KNOCKING AT THE GATE OF LIFE

AND OTHER HEALING EXERCISES FROM CHINA

KNOCKING
AT THE
GATE OF
LIFE

AND OTHER
HEALING
EXERCISES
FROM CHINA

The Official Handbook of the People's Republic of China

Translated by Edward C. Chang, Ph.D., Chairman
Departments of Psychology, Sociology and Social Work
Albany State College, Albany, Georgia

Foreword by Haig Ignatius, M.D., Dipl.Ac. (NCCA), M.Ac. (U.K.),
Vice President and Senior Faculty, Traditional Acupuncture Institute

 Rodale Press, Emmaus, Pennsylvania

Printed in the United States of America

Book design by Anita Noble
Illustrations by Susan Rosenberger
Book layout by Jane C. Knutila

Library of Congress Cataloging in Publication Data

Cho, Ta-hung.
 Knocking at the gate of life and other healing exercises from China.

  Translation of: I liao t'i yü ch'ang shih.
  Includes index.
  1. Exercise therapy.   I. Chang, Edward C.
RM725.C456313 1985   615.8'2   85–14297
ISBN 0-87857-581-2 hardcover
ISBN 0-87857-582-0 paperback
2 4 6 8 10 9 7 5 3 1   hardcover
2 4 6 8 10 9 7 5 3 1   paperback

To all those interested in the Chinese way to healing—
康 , the symbol for health

Contents

Acknowledgments

I am grateful for the encouragement or assistance of many people. I wish particularly to thank Dr. Isaiah Azariah, Dr. M. B. Bowman, Dr. Wilbur Thomas and Kathy Nulty for reviewing portions of the manuscript. Dr. Samuel Masih made my job easier by helping me with the use of a word processor.

My special appreciation is given to Mimi, Norman and Emily for doing my share of the household responsibilities and for leaving me alone so that I could concentrate on my work during weekends and evening hours. They have been my source of inspiration.

I want to thank all those at Rodale Press who took part, small or big, in the production of this book. I especially want to express my appreciation to Mark Bricklin and John Feltman for their encouragement and support. Rich Huttner, Bill Gottlieb, Debora Tkac, Jerry O'Brien, Karen Schell, Anita Noble and Jane Knutila all contributed. Nor would I want to forget Sue Lagler, Roberta Mulliner and Dorothy Smickley.

I wish to thank my editor Nona Cleland for her continuous support, encouragement and inspiration. Her editorial acumen and skill have turned this into a "real book."

Gratitude also goes to Daniel Kinderlehrer, M.D., who read this manuscript and offered a number of valuable suggestions for its improvement.

This list would not be complete without thanks to Susan Rosenberger for her beautiful work with the illustrations.

Finally, I owe a special debt of gratitude to Dr. Cho Ta Hung without whose original work this translation would not have been possible.

Edward C. Chang, Ph.D.

Foreword

Since President John F. Kennedy's encouragement of physical fitness to improve the nation's health, we have seen increasing numbers of people commit themselves to doing exercises: running, jogging, swimming and cycling; then adding mechanical exercises — weight machines, stationary bicycles, mini-trampolines, rowing machines and even gyms in homes and offices.

However, the percentage of the population that exercises is still relatively small and represents mostly the vigorous young and middle-aged. Some special exercises are prescribed for pregnancy, obesity, heart conditions, back problems and other musculoskeletal conditions, but it is mainly healthy and vigorous people who are exercising — doing exercises preventively to maintain their already good physical health.

It was with these observations in mind that I noticed, during a visit to China in 1982, that in the early morning hours, the streets of Kun Ming were filled with people. Some were running, some doing calisthenics of various kinds, some doing *Tai Chi* movements, some exercising in groups, but most of them were doing individual exercises, each different from the other.

People swarmed at the gate of a park on a lakeside, awaiting the 6 A.M. opening of the gate, then entering with a pass or by paying a small fee. Little did I then know they were not just doing the same "morning constitutionals" that we do here in America. They were really *knocking at the gate of life* as they entered the park, for they exercised to improve their body-mind-spirits.

Not only were the large numbers of people so remarkable, and the individually different exercises they did, but the range of ages impressed me. Little children often did things in groups. Elderly people, some obviously frail, were out there in the early morning. Some ran in pairs or did gymnastics together.

Later in the day, at the times we would think of as our coffee breaks or lunch breaks, people in schools, hospitals and other buildings emptied out into the courtyards or nearby fields and began exercising. Most of them exercised in groups, some playing basketball, some doing calisthenics, some *Tai Chi* in a group, and some, their own individual exercise.

As I came to understand their medical tradition, I realized that acupuncture was only a small part of what is now called "Traditional Chinese Medicine," or TCM. This medical tradition has always included herbal remedies, acupuncture and moxibustion, manipulation, dietary regimens, breathing exercises and physical exercises. Attitudinal or meditative techniques are incorporated with the breathing and physical exercises.

With these methods, many of what we call "chronic conditions" are treated or ameliorated with the use of little or no medications or drugs. In this book, when the medical treatment for specific conditions is discussed, there are often recommendations for exercises, massage and manipulative techniques as part of the treatment regimen.

This is the first book in English that I have found to be so comprehensive in this regard. Written in China by Dr. Cho Ta Hung, and translated by Dr. Edward Chang of Albany State College in Georgia, it discusses the seven categories of exercises; the advantages, precautions or even dangers of each exercise; the conditions and organs that benefit from the exercise; and sometimes the energetic meridians that are affected to improve the condition.

The exercises are described very specifically. There are very gentle exercises—movements of the toes or fingers or the "gaze of the eyes"—accompanied by mental attitudes and breathing exercises. And there are vigorous exercises, some including imagery—as when mimicking a monkey, bear or tiger. The author occasionally includes massage of certain acupuncture points, hot or cold water baths and even air baths and sunbaths.

The descriptions include movements of the tongue, tapping of the teeth, self-massage with "knocking" techniques, mental attitudes and imagery—"pushing mountains," for instance. Gymnastics and group sports are recommended for some patients—including those with paralysis. The body-mind connection is often brought forth. You might even think of many of these exercises as a sort of physical meditation.

An exercise may be preventive or may stop the progression of an existing disease. It may help reduce the amount of medication as it decreases the discomforts of a particular problem. The exercise may also mean improvement or, at times, actual clearing of an illness completely.

This book gives the patient an opportunity to participate directly in the treatment of his or her illness. It encourages optimism about solving physical problems.

A variety of conditions, including every physiological system in the body, is covered. Among the many specific conditions are myopia, nerve deafness, hepatitis, hypertension, periartenitis, coronary disease, Buerger's disease, dysmenorrhea, pregnancy, prostatitis, digestive disorders, postural (scoliosis) and arthritic conditions, knee-cap strain, hemorrhoids, skin and hair problems, sweating of hands and feet, emphysema, silicosis, pigeon-breast, asthma, epilepsy, flatfeet—and many more. Paralysis (hemiplegia and paraplegia) is dealt with so that a patient can learn to get up and stand at the bedside.

In the discussion of many of these conditions, the pathophysiology of the illness is also described, so that one has a sense of what the exercise is actually doing for the patient.

As a physician-acupuncturist, I see that the exercises are designed to modify or improve the energetics of various body-mind functions. The concept of the *energetic physiology* of the body has always been a fundamental aspect of Oriental medical science, just as *biochemical and cellular physiology* have been in Western medical science.

I admire the clarity and attention to detail, as well as the comprehensive scope, of Dr. Cho's book. Dr. Chang's translation is to be commended for the accuracy with which he has captured its healing spirit.

Knocking at the Gate of Life has something to offer most everyone—young and old, vigorous or weak, the anxious and the contented. It is a marvelous manual for the layperson, healthy or not, and offers treatment recommendations useful for health practitioners of every modality I can imagine. To name just a few, I would mention the massage and physical therapist, acupuncturist, ophthalmologist, gynecologist, internist, urologist, orthopedic surgeon, neurologist and certainly the psychiatrist.

I know you, the reader, will enjoy many of the descriptions in this book. And as you read, you'll recognize how you or people you know would benefit from a particular exercise. I challenge you—the one now holding this book in your hands—to find the exercise that is best for you.

In the tradition of the Far East, this book offers an opportunity to the West—to knock at the gate of life!

Haig Ignatius, M.D., Dipl.Ac. (NCCA),
    M.Ac. (U.K.)
Vice President and Senior Faculty of the
    Traditional Acupuncture Institute
March, 1985

CHAPTER ONE

An Introduction to Healing Exercise

康

Wherever you go in China during the morning hours, you will see men and women doing healing exercises to protect or restore their health.

What is healing exercise? It's simply exercise that has been shown to have significant therapeutic value. It can both treat *and* prevent certain diseases.

Healing exercise differs from regular exercise and other therapeutic techniques in several ways. First, healing exercise is designed primarily for, but not necessarily limited to, people who are sick or physically weak. It's used, for instance, to treat patients who suffer from chronic illnesses.

The nature of the illness and the patient's condition and habits determine the type of exercise to be used. And individual exercises may be modified to suit special needs, preferably under the guidance of a health professional. The elderly and the physically weak will find these exercises particularly useful in improving their condition.

Healing exercise also differs from other therapeutic techniques because it does not rely on drugs, medicine or surgery. Instead, healing exercise is designed to build up the patient's physical strength and improve his or her physiological functioning.

Healing exercise frequently involves the coordination of mind and body. That's why *Ch'i Kung* (The Art of Breathing) and *Tai Chi Chuan* (Supreme Ultimate Exercise) are especially effective in treating diseases that are closely linked to the emotions such as colitis, depression, hypertension and peptic ulcers.

The Development of Healing Exercise in China

Although the coinage "healing exercise" is relatively recent, the use of physical exercise as a therapeutic technique can be traced to about 1000 B.C. in China. The ancient Chinese probably accidentally discovered the value of massage and exercise in relieving pain and improving joint motion as they engaged in physical labor and rubbed and pressed muscles that became sore.

Even earlier—in the period of T'an Yao (2360 B.C.), people used dancing as a form of therapy for arthritis. Later, during the Warring Period (403–221 B.C.), *Dao Yin* (psychophysiological exercise) and *Ta Na* (breathing exercise) were introduced by the Taoists as effective techniques for the prevention and treatment of certain ailments. Remnants of embroidered silk showing different postures used in meditation and exercise, unearthed recently with other artifacts by archaeologists in Changsha, China, attest to the antiquity of therapeutic exercise in China.

Toward the end of the Han Dynasty, a medical specialist named Hua To (A.D. 141–203) advocated physical exercise to improve resistance to disease. His system of healing is called *Wu Chin Hsi* (Five Animal Play). It imitates the movement of tigers, deer, bears, monkeys and birds. Later *Tai Chi Chuan* (Supreme Ultimate Exercise), *Pa Tuan Chin* (The Eight Sets of Embroidery), and *Shih Erh Tuan Chin* (The Twelve Sets of Embroidery) were invented and became popular among the ordinary people. These exercises were found to be very effective in preventing disease. Such documents as *Nei Ching* (The Classic of Internal Medicine) and *Tsien Chin Fang* (The Thousand Prescriptions) chronicle the history and how-to's of healing exercises.

The Forms and Methods of Healing Exercise

Healing exercise may be divided into seven categories: therapeutic gymnastics, exercise therapy, mechanical therapy, *Ch'i Kung* (The Art of Breathing), *An Mu* (massage), nature's treatment—water showers or baths at various temperatures, air baths and sunbaths—and finally, recreational exercise.

Therapeutic gymnastics: Of all the types of healing exercises, therapeutic gymnastics deserves special attention because of its effectiveness. Each exercise has a purpose and is specially chosen to help heal specific diseases. For example, the therapeutic gymnastics for chronic bronchitis will probably differ from those meant for relieving pain in the waist and leg. By the same token, exercises for high blood pressure are quite unlike those for treating emphysema.

A therapeutic gymnastics session usually consists of 5 to 20 series of exercises. Each of the series calls for special preparation, posture, exercise content and number of repetitions. Emphasis should, however, be placed on quality of the exercise rather than its quantity or variety. Sometimes the same healing results can be achieved by a few repetitions of the most effective exercises.

Exercise therapy: Exercise therapy can help prevent and treat certain illnesses. It includes *Tai Chi Chuan,* various gymnastic exercises, walking, hiking, canoeing, taking field trips and other less rigorous sports. Generally speaking, exercise therapy is more effective than therapeutic gymnastics in improving the function of the heart

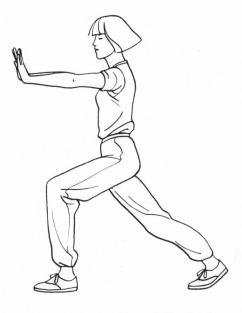

Figure 2. *Exercise therapy*

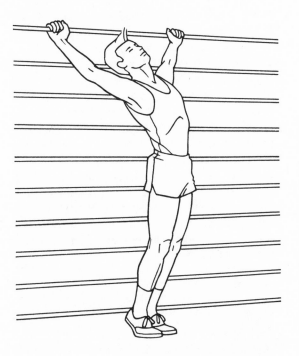

Figure 1. *Therapeutic gymnastics*

and lungs. Exercise therapy is most appropriate for patients who suffer from chronic illnesses if they have the physical strength.

Therapy with mechanical aids: This method calls for special exercise equipment. Its aim is to restore the normal function of the limbs and joints and to help correct any deformities. Exercise bicycles, for example, can help strengthen leg muscles. Or, using a specially constructed wheel, they can enhance the function of shoulder joints.

Ch'i Kung: Ch'i Kung combines mental concentration with breathing exercise. It is designed to cultivate and nourish *ch'i,* or energy flow, within the body. The Chinese have found that *Ch'i Kung* is an effective healer of many chronic

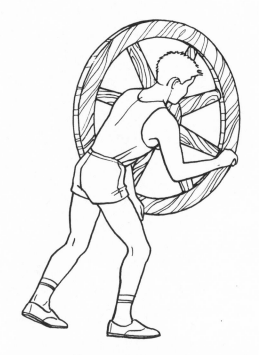

Figure 3. *Therapy with mechanical aids*

diseases, including depression, high blood pressure, peptic ulcer and duodenitis (inflammation of a portion of the small intestine).

An Mu: An Mu (massage) can be done by the patient or by a health professional. It can ease pain, stimulate blood and lymphatic circulation, increase muscle flexibility, accelerate digestion, reduce fatigue and relax muscles.

Nature's treatment: Water, sunlight and fresh air can enhance your health when these elements are used with other forms of healing exercise.

Recreational exercise: Recreational activities such as gardening, knitting and other do-it-yourself hobbies can not only develop muscles but also relax the nervous system. They are an excellent way to encourage an adequate amount of physical activity which helps promote physical and psychological fitness.

No healing exercise or physical therapy can be considered a panacea. Like any other therapeutic technique, each has limitations. One may be particularly useful for certain ailments, but have only minimal or secondary effects on others. Chinese doctors have found healing exercise most effective for treating the following types of diseases:

• Chronic diseases associated with the respiratory, digestive, cardiovascular and reproductive systems. Therapeutic exercise has proven effective in the treatment of pulmonary tuberculosis, emphysema, chronic tracheitis, bronchial asthma, chronic constipation, hemorrhoids, prolapse of the anus, gastroptosis (fallen stomach), high blood pressure and prolapse of the uterus. It also can be used to treat depression and arthritis. It works because it helps improve the function of internal organs, increases immunity to disease, relieves symptoms and inhibits further progress of the disease.

• Paralysis resulting from nerve injury or impaired blood flow through cerebral vessels.

• Stiff joints due to external injury or to arthritis.

• Abnormal posture, such as curvature of the spine, or other structural problems may be correctable to some degree—even flatfeet if the case is not too severe.

Healing Exercise Is Valuable

Healing exercise helps to cure disease. Both repeated scientific experiments and patients who have used these exercises testify to this.

Therapeutic exercise effectively prevents and treats diseases by correcting a number of problems. Some diseases stem from work habits. For instance, a person who works at a desk most of the time and doesn't often move will have slack abdominal muscles and weakened intestines. Chronic constipation may develop.

Other people may develop neurasthenia, a common mental and physical condition characterized by lethargy, depression, fatigue and sometimes insomnia, because of their concentration on mental activity without any form of physical exertion. Of course, a balance between mental and physical activities should be the goal.

Diseases triggered by weaknesses of the heart and lungs—emphysema and chronic circulatory problems, for example—can be helped by healing exercises. Both lungs and heart, respiratory and circulatory functions, will grow stronger. Eventually all symptoms may subside.

Medications are needed for such diseases as tuberculosis, high blood pressure and diabetes when those diseases have reached a critical stage. But if the patient's organs are too weak, or their function is too ineffectual to respond, drug therapy may not be adequate. But regular healing exercise can strengthen the internal organs and increase the efficiency of the metabolic process, making it easier for the body to readily respond to the medication. For this reason healing exercise can have secondary benefits in the treatment of these diseases.

Some patients who suffer from chronic diseases have become so accustomed to a passive life that they have lost the desire to engage in almost any form of physical activity. As a result, the physiological function of their bodies tends to become weak. The effect of a lack of exercise over a prolonged period of time may show up in symptoms such as depression, difficulty in breathing, circulatory problems, weak heart, problems with digestion, metabolic imbalance, muscle tightness and even shrinkage of muscles. With these conditions, the patient may be vulnerable to other diseases in addition to finding recovery difficult from the original problem. But the patient can help the recovery process greatly by doing exercises that will improve the performance of major internal organs, help regulate respiratory and blood circulation and revitalize the digestive system. These exercises can help regain lost health.

Some diseases are primarily related to the impairment of body movement such as joint immobility, consolidation or stiffening or muscular paralysis. Such impairments can be helped by proper exercise. Gymnastics can improve joint

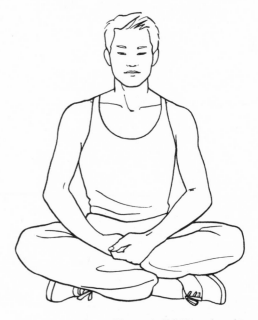

Figure 4. Ch'i Kung *breathing*

mobility, strengthen nerves and muscles and help to regain control of muscular movement.

More Reasons for Doing Healing Exercise

Chairman Mao Tse-tung was a strong advocate of the use of physical exercise to improve the health of the Chinese people. He encouraged all kinds of physical activity, including gymnastics, competitive sports, jogging, hiking, swimming and *Tai Chi Chuan*. Under his patronage, China made significant progress in developing the techniques involved in healing exercises.

Some might ask why patients should exercise when medicine can do the job. Questions such as this come up especially in light of the tremendous advances in modern medicine. But healing exercise has a unique therapeutic value not present in other kinds of treatment. Although many chronic diseases can be helped by medicine alone, therapeutic exercise can make recovery and restoration of normal health faster. Clinical experience has revealed that medicine alone does not solve most problems. But when medicine is used with healing exercise, one can enhance the other. The benefit to the patient may be decisive.

The advantages of healing exercise are numerous. For one, it is easy to do. It's also cost-free because it involves no special facilities. Its therapeutic effects are obvious. Following are some of the benefits of doing therapeutic exercise on a regular and systematic basis:

• Therapeutic exercise helps proper function of the heart, lungs and joints. It also promotes muscular development that cannot be achieved by pharmacotherapy.

• Healing exercise is a holistic therapy. Unlike other therapies that focus only on the affected part, exercise treats the entire body by toning the

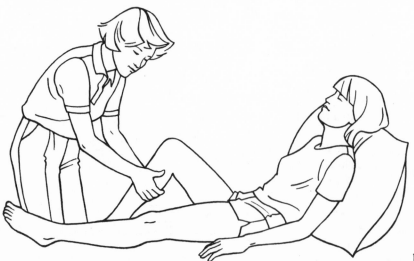

Figure 5. An Mu *(massage)*

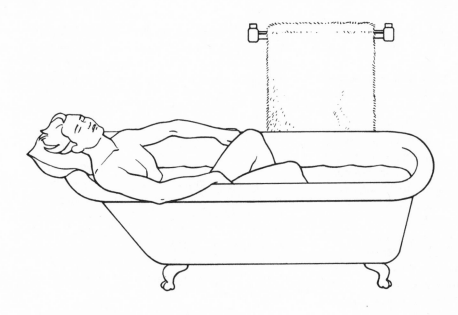

Figure 6. *Water therapy*

nervous system and the circulation of the blood. It also improves the body's ability to absorb and transport nutrients, thereby increasing immunity.

• Healing exercise is a form of self-therapy. The patient must actively participate in the treatment process. Since personal involvement can make a big difference, the patient is more inclined to develop a positive attitude toward the treatment and confidence in his or her power to affect the outcome. All of this can hasten recovery.

• Exercise is a natural therapy. It relies upon the ability of everyone—male and female, young and old—to do exercises. And there are no negative side effects if the methods are followed correctly.

• It's a preventive technique. Prevention, of course, is better than cure. Generally speaking, diseases can be attributed to both external and, even more significantly, to internal factors. If we can improve our physical strength and increase our bodies' ability to resist diseases, we may be less susceptible to sickness despite external factors. We all know that in similar circumstances some people get sick easily, while others remain healthy. This is because the healthy persons have acquired the ability to resist the invasion of disease-producing agents by taking care of their internal conditions. Healing exercise places great importance on preventing disease.

Develop a Routine for Your Healing Exercise

In order to get the desired results, you must do your healing exercises on a regular basis. The reason is very simple: it takes time to increase muscular strength, enhance joint motion and improve the functioning of heart and lungs. Improvement is gradual and proportional to the time spent in practice.

So it's important for persons who want to engage in healing exercise to practice regularly and continuously over a long period of time. A gradual and systematic program will bring the best possible results. In the early stages, exercises should proceed slowly from simple to complex techniques and from easier to more strenuous patterns. In brief, the whole treatment process should be well planned and systematic.

Any male over 35 or female over 40 who has a previously sedentary lifestyle should consult with his or her physician before embarking on any exercise program. In particular, people at risk of developing coronary artery disease may need to undergo a cardiac stress test. This will determine that exercise is safe to do or the limits

at which exercise can be done safely. Risk factors for coronary artery disease include hypertension, diabetes, smoking, elevated cholesterol levels or a close family member with a history of heart disease.

No Exercise during Fever

It is not advisable to exercise when you have a fever. Engaging in physical exercise during fever may have harmful effects on the body, particularly if the exercise is strenuous. First of all, the body obviously produces extra heat during fever. If you exercise at this time, the increased metabolic reactions and heat production aggravated by exercise will raise your body temperature so much that it may be harmful.

During fever, proteins within the tissues are undergoing chemical changes while vitamins are being consumed quickly. Doing exercise at this time will increase metabolism and negatively affect your ability to resist disease. In addition, for each one-degree increase in body temperature on the Celsius scale, the heart will beat 10 to 20 extra times per minute. Cardiac output during fever may put a strain on the heart. Engaging in strenuous physical exercise at this time will place an even greater burden on the heart and may lead to heart malfunctioning.

Finally, it is important to remember that fever frequently is symptomatic of certain contagious diseases in their early stages. A person really needs plenty of rest rather than physical exercise at such times.

Though it is not advisable to engage in healing exercise when you have fever, a chronic disease patient may do *some* walking and practice *Ch'i Kung* if the fever is of very low grade.

But remember, physical exercise may do

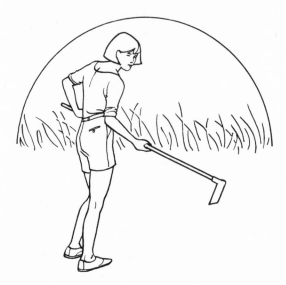

Figure 7. *Recreational exercise*

more harm than good during the critical stage of a disease. It might cause other complications such as rupture of an aneurysm—a bulge in the wall of a vein, artery or the heart.

How to Self-Monitor Your Healing Exercise Program

Since healing exercise is simple and easy to do, chronic patients may, on the advice of their doctor, practice therapeutic exercise in the hospital or clinic, at home or even in school under the supervision of a health teacher. However, it is also necessary for patients to monitor their own progress.

Self-monitoring simply means observing your own body reactions during exercise in order to make necessary adjustments in intensity, style and method. The intensity of therapeutic exercise may be arbitrarily divided into three levels according to the pulse rate measured immediately after exercise. An average adult, who normally has a pulse rate somewhere between 60 and 80 beats per minute, may see it increase to 120–140 after very rigorous exercise, or to 90–110 following heavy exercise. If the exercise is less rigorous, the pulse rate may remain the same or only exceed the normal pulse by 10 beats per minute. The pulse rate during healing exercise is usually below 110.

If any of the following symptoms are observed after exercise, practice should be discontinued: fever, insomnia, loss of weight, feeling of fatigue, worsening of illness or any painful sensation or swelling in the body. It is possible that these symptoms might have been caused by rigorous exercise or by not correctly following instructions. If you develop any of these symptoms it is advisable to have a medical examination or to ask an experienced teacher of physical education to help you determine the cause. It is very important to self-monitor your exercise program so that problems can be immediately identified and corrective action taken. Self-monitoring is a sound practice and a good precaution.

Healing Exercise at School

Healing exercise is useful not only in hospitals, clinics and in homes, but also in schools. Children with chronic ailments or physical disabilities can be grouped together for preventive and therapeutic exercises.

Children who need healing physical education classes can be classified into two groups—the chronically ill and the physically handicapped. The first should consist of children who suffer from heart diseases, pulmonary tuberculosis, gastric ulcer, duodenal ulcer, rheumatoid arthritis, emotional and behavioral problems, and anemia. This group shouldn't be larger than 15 children. The second group of children, those suffering from infantile paralysis, spinal malformation and other joint problems, should not be larger than 10.

The group with chronic diseases will follow the teacher doing healing exercises such as *Tai Chi Chuan,* gymnastics and games such as badminton, basketball and volleyball. The physically impaired group may need individual guidance in corrective exercises for the first few lessons before practicing individually.

More Ways to Help Yourself Heal

Therapeutic exercise improves physical strength, helps the body to build up immunity and enables it to combat existing disease. But although some chronic patients understand the healing value of exercise, they pay less attention to other important health factors such as eating, sleeping and the psychological aspects of living.

The fact of the matter is that healing exercise is by no means a panacea, nor should it be treated as an isolated phenomenon. It should be accompanied by other forms of treatment.

First of all, chronic patients should develop an optimistic spirit when it comes to combating disease. Patients who anticipate fighting a losing battle may be too worried to achieve any significant results even if they do exercise.

Those who are sick should work on a correct attitude toward medication. Some patients have too much faith in therapeutic exercise and reject medicine. On the other hand, some may rely on medicine so much that they fail to see the value of other techniques. Both extremes should be avoided.

Medication may be necessary for treating both acute and chronic diseases during the developmental stage. And it is sometimes also necessary for patients to resort to medication later even though they do healing exercise. Medicine may be reduced or eventually discontinued only after the problem has been relieved as a result of regular exercise.

Those who are ill should pay special attention to the kind of food and drink they consume. Good nutrition comes from eating a variety of foods, and it need not cost a lot. Some people wrongly assume that nutritional value and the cost of food must necessarily be correlated. As a matter of fact, vegetables and some other less expensive edibles may actually have higher nutritional value than a rich costly diet. What is most important is to have a balanced diet. Eat a variety of foods, without concentrating on a few. The elderly and the physically weak should try to eat more vegetables, which are particularly wholesome and health-giving.

Patients should also keep a balance between work and recreation, adhere to a regular bedtime and set aside a particular time for exercise. In short, follow a regular routine.

Patients who have chronic diseases must cut down on smoking and drinking alcohol. Smoking and alcohol consumption have been found to impede the treatment of disease. Patients who avoid smoking and alcohol and who follow a regular exercise program benefit the most from physical exercise therapy.

CHAPTER TWO

Healing Exercises for Everyone

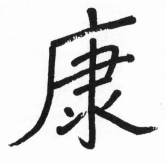

No matter if you're 90 or 9, a weight lifter or too weak to lift your arm, there are Chinese healing exercises for you. Exercises that will make you feel more alive when you wake up in the morning and exercises that will help you sleep better at night. Designed to strengthen and build disease-fighting resistance in people who are healthy, many of the exercises in this chapter can also help those suffering from nagging chronic diseases.

The Twelve Sets of Embroidery, Five Animal Play—such poetic-sounding exercises have been treasured, practiced and polished over centuries. They come to you with a long history of healing, blessed by the affections of millions of people. Others, equally cherished, are as modern as the jogger on your corner.

Five Animal Play

Wu Chin Hsi, Five Animal Play, was developed by Hua To, a famous Chinese doctor of the later

Han Dynasty. The exercise consists of movements that mimic the gestures and mannerisms of five different animals. You will imitate the fierce and untamed tiger and the graceful-necked deer. You'll also walk steadily and lumber like a bear, move adroitly like a monkey and stretch your arms like a flying bird.

For his time, Hua To was pragmatic and empirical in his approach to medicine. He was against superstition and attacked the Confucianism-oriented medical theory built on supernaturalism. His Five Animal Play was based on his belief that exercise and medicine could be integrated in developing physical fitness and preventing and fighting against disease. He developed his exercises more than a thousand years before the same idea was conceived in Sweden.

Many variations of the Five Animal Play have been added since Hua To's time. The original movements have been continuously modified and improved. One variety that is easy to learn and is known to have good results is presented in the following section. You may practice the whole set or choose part of it, depending on your condition.

Bear Play

1. Stand with your feet a shoulder width apart and your arms hanging naturally. (See Fig. 8a.) Breathe in and out deeply 3 to 5 times. Then sway your waist, hips and groin in a natural but bearlike way.

2. Bend your right knee slightly and swing your right shoulder downward to the front with your arm hanging naturally. At the same time, turn your left shoulder slightly backward and lift your left hand slightly. (See Fig. 8b.)

3. Reverse the position in step 2. Bend your left knee down to the front with your arm hanging

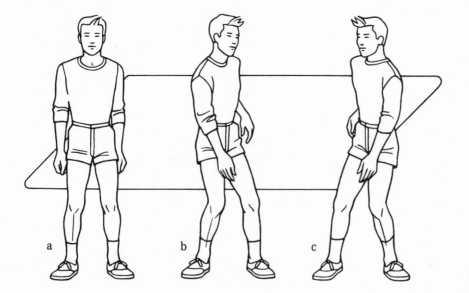

a   b   c

Figure 8. *Bear play*

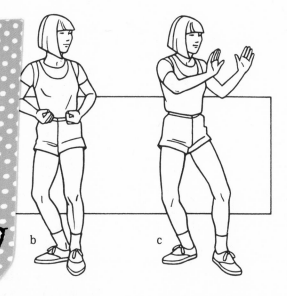

Figure 9. *Tiger play*

right shoulder slightly
hand slightly. (See

many times as you
joint mobility and the
and stomach.

principles for mimicking

waist and swaying

relax and move your

dy in setting your feet on

and thoughtful while focusing your
attention on *Tan Tien* (Cinnabar Field, the area
located about 3 inches below your navel).

Tiger Play

1. Let your arms hang down naturally. Keep
your neck straight and your face relaxed. Look
straight ahead. Keep your mouth closed with
your tongue gently touching the roof of your
mouth. Do not bow or thrust your chest foward.
Move your heels together to form a 90-degree
angle. This is basically a standing-at-attention
posture, but you are to relax your entire body.
(See Fig. 9a.) Stand in this position for a few
moments.

2. Slowly bend your knees to lower your
body. With your weight on your right leg, lift
your left heel slightly off the ground and bring it
close to your right ankle. At the same time, form
fists and bring them to the sides of your waist
with the fingers facing up. With your eyes, look
toward the left. (See Fig. 9b.)

3. Then take one step forward to the left.
Keep your right foot half a step behind. The
distance between your heels should be about 12
inches. Keep your weight on your right foot. At
the same time, lift your fists toward your chest
with the fingers facing your body. As your fists
approach the level of your mouth, turn your fists

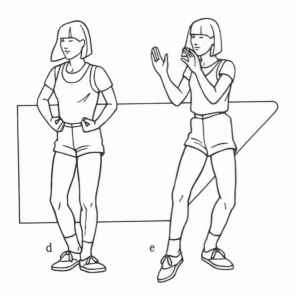

Figure 9. *Tiger play*

Monkey Play

1. Stand for a few minutes as if at attention but relaxed as for tiger play.

2. Bend your knees slowly to lower your body. Step forward gracefully with your left foot. At the same time, raise your left hand up beside your chest. As soon as it reaches the level of your mouth, make it into a claw and thrust it forward as if you were reaching out to grasp an object. (See Fig. 10a.)

3. Then step forward with your right foot and lift your left heel slightly off the ground. At the same time raise your right hand up beside your chest. When your hand is level with your mouth, thrust it forward in a clawlike position with your wrist bent. Bring your left hand back to your side with the elbow bent. (See Fig. 10b.)

over, open your hands and push out strongly at chest level with your palms open. Your "tigers' mouths"—the space between your thumbs and forefingers—will be facing each other. Look at the tip of your left index finger with both eyes. (See Fig. 9c.)

4. Repeat this same exercise to the right. Starting again from the at-attention position, bend your knees, put your weight on your left leg, lift your right heel off the ground and bring it close to your left ankle. Proceed with the exercise as in steps 2 and 3 except that your direction is to the right. (See Fig. 9d and e.)

You can repeat the sequence as many times as you like. In doing the exercise, try to capture the fighting spirit of a tiger and to imitate its quickness and grace. Be composed yet fierce.

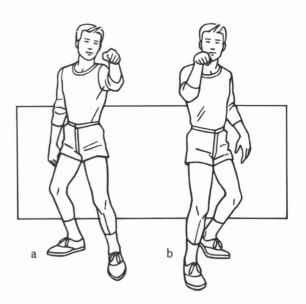

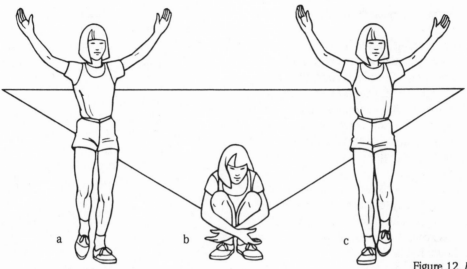

Figure 12. *Bird play*

Strengthening with *Yee Chin Ching*

Yee Chin Ching was a popular fitness method in ancient China. Many centuries have passed, but the popularity of this exercise has not faded with time. Many people today practice *Yee Chin Ching* as part of their physical conditioning, and it is especially popular among traditional Chinese doctors who specialize in therapies based on postural alignment and massage and who do this exercise themselves.

The practice of *Yee Chin Ching* not only helps promote good health and develops physical fitness and strength, but it also can be used as part of the recovery program of people suffering from bone-related ailments. It is especially effective at increasing muscular strength.

It is believed that *Yee Chin Ching* was orig-

inally developed for training muscles and the tissues that line and connect muscles, the fascia. Literally *yee* means "transformation"; *chin*, "muscle"; and *ching*, "method." *Yee Chin Ching* is thus a method for transforming weak slack muscles into strong solid ones.

The movements of *Yee Chin Ching* are hard and forceful. But in hardness there lies softness. In motion, there is placidness. In *Yee Chin Ching*, *yi*—consciousness—and force are united.

The movements of *Yee Chin Ching* are similar to those of *Pa Tuan Chin,* but *Yee Chin* exceeds *Pa Tuan Chin* in both demands on strength and rigors of movement.

During *Yee Chin,* you must maintain a tranquil mind, a composed mental spirit and a harmonious breathing rhythm. In addition, you must attempt to unite external force with internal force and motion with placidness.

The following describes one set of *Yee Chin Ching.*

Form 1. Folding hands in front of chest: Stand with your feet a shoulder width apart and your arms hanging naturally at your sides. Keep your back straight. Focus your eyes on distant objects and direct your full concentration on them.

1. Leading with the backs of your open hands, raise your arms straight out in front of you, stopping at shoulder level. Your palms should be facing down.

2. Turn your palms over to face each other and draw them slowly to a distance of about one fist away from your chest. Your fingertips should just touch and your palms should be facing your chest as shown in Fig. 13a.

Remember that this form is the starting position. Attention should be paid to three things: your body should be kept in a natural and comfortable position, your mind should be kept free of distracting thoughts, and you should mentally concentrate. Also keep your breathing natural.

Form 2. Raising arms to form a carrying pole: Begin in the standard relaxed, upright position, your feet a shoulder width apart.

1. Grasp the ground with your toes. Turn your palms to face out to the sides.

2. As you rise on your toes, lift your arms straight out to the sides to shoulder level. Your palms should be up. (See Fig. 13b.) Now sink back down on your feet, let your arms fall and relax.

Remember to move your arms and rise on your toes simultaneously. Keep your mental focus on your palms and toes. Breathe in and out freely.

Form 3. Holding the sky up with both hands: Assume the starting posture, standing straight, feet as wide apart as your shoulders.

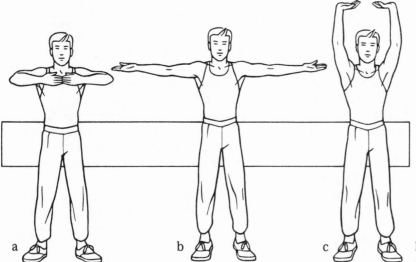

a   b   c

Figure 13. Yee Chin Ching
strengthening exercises

1. Raise both arms slowly out toward your sides with your palms facing up. Stretch them over your head, palms still up, fingers pointing inward and just touching as if you were holding up the sky. At the same time, lift your heels slightly off the ground, clench your teeth, touch your tongue to the roof of your mouth, and breathe deeply. Mentally concentrate on your hands. (See Fig. 13c.)

2. Make your hands into fists and lower your arms from over your head to shoulder level out to the sides. At the same time, allow your heels to sink to the floor. You should move slowly, but with muscular tension in your arms.

Remember to mentally look at your hands — don't actually look at them with your eyes. The movements of Form 1 to Form 3 follow each other and should be performed consecutively. Do each form only once.

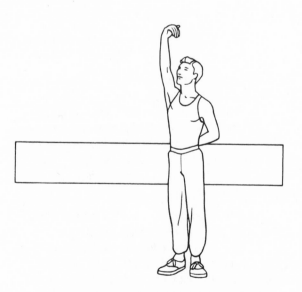

Figure 14. *Exchanging one star for another*

Form 4. Exchanging one star for another: Continue from the preceding form. Stand with feet apart and your arms out sideways at shoulder level.

1. Raise your right hand slowly over your head. Turn your palm over so that it faces down. Bring your fingers close to each other and curl your fingertips slightly down. Lift your head and look at your right palm as you lower your left hand and put it, palm facing out, behind your waist. (See Fig. 14.) Hold this pose for 3 to 5 deep breaths.

2. Raise your left hand over your head to the same position as you did your right at the same time as you are lowering the left to the behind-the-waist position. Breathe in and out 3 to 5 times in this position.

Do 3 to 5 complete repetitions of this exercise.

During this exercise, look at your lifted hand, but focus your attention on the back of your waist where your other hand is. Breathe in and out through your nose or breathe in through your nose and out through your mouth. As you inhale, press the back of your waist gently with the rear of your hand. Release the press as you exhale. Your breathing should be even and slow.

Form 5. Pulling the cow's tail backward: Continue from the pose that ended the last form.

1. Withdraw your right hand from the rear of your waist and stretch it forward, turning it palm down. When your hand reaches shoulder level, bend your elbow slightly and bring your fingers together to form a "plum flower"—curl your fingers slightly in. Now take a long step forward with your right leg. Bend your right knee while keeping the left leg straight to form a sort of arch. At the same time, lower the left

hand, form it into a loose fist and draw it slightly to the rear of your left hip. (See Fig. 15.)

2. As you inhale, put your focus on your right hand and think of it as if it were pulling a cow's tail backward. During your exhalation, put your attention on your left hand as though it were drawing the cow forward. Breathe in and out in this manner. Notice that your imaginary pulling backward and drawing forward are creating tension on your legs, trunk, shoulders and elbows—and they're meant to.

3. Alternate the position of your left leg with your right leg. With your left foot now in front, lift your left hand forward and form a "plum flower." Draw your right hand backward in a loose fist as in step 1.

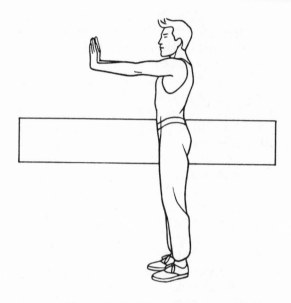

Figure 16. *Pushing palms out to stretch arms*

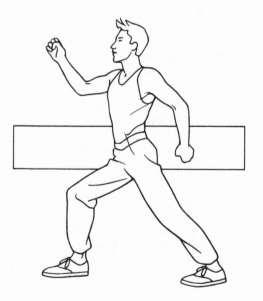

Figure 15. *Pulling the cow's tail backward*

4. Inhale and exhale, again pulling and drawing on the cow's tail.

Repeat the entire exercise 3 to 5 times.

Remember to keep your mental focus on each hand in turn, but look straight ahead. As you breathe, remember to keep your lower abdomen comfortable and relaxed. The force should be in your arms.

Form 6. Pushing palms out to stretch arms: Start from the ending position of the previous form. Draw your right foot forward to line up with your left foot, and stand up straight. Place both hands in front of your chest with your palms wide open and facing out and your fingers straight up.

1. Make "mountain-pushing" palms with your hands by keeping them at 90-degree angles to your wrist, palms facing out. Push out slowly from your chest with increasing force until your arms are fully extended. Keep your entire body straight, your eyes wide open and your gaze on distant objects. (See Fig. 16.)

2. Slowly return your hands to the position in front of your chest.

Repeat this exercise 3 to 5 times.

Remember to exert force gradually. When your palms reach their full extension, the force is almost powerful enough to push down the imaginary mountain. This is why the hand position is called a "mountain-pushing" palm. You should also keep your breathing rhythm harmonious. Exhale while pushing forward, and inhale while bringing the hands back.

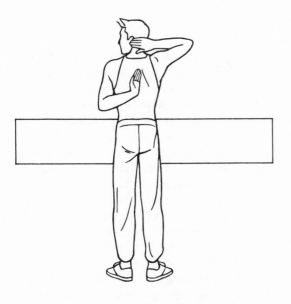

Figure 17. *Drawing a sword*

Form 7. Drawing a sword: Start from the previous form with your arms extended at shoulder level and your palms in the "mountain-pushing" position.

1. Then clasp the rear of your head with your right hand. Pull on your left ear gently while keeping your elbow back. Turn your head to the left while putting your left hand down between your shoulder blades as far as possible with your palm out. (See Fig. 17.)

2. While breathing in, reach behind your head with your right hand and tug and squeeze your left ear, keeping your elbow back and your neck straight. Concentrate on your right elbow. Breathe out and relax. Breathe in and out in this position 3 to 5 times.

3. Raise your right hand up and put it between your shoulder blades. At the same time, put the palm of your left hand to the rear of your head. Pull your right ear gently with your fingers. Keep your elbow back and your head turned right.

4. While breathing in, squeeze and pull on your right ear with your hand. Keep your left elbow pulled back and your attention focused on it. Relax and exhale. Breathe in and out and repeat your ear pulling and elbow stretching.

Repeat this exercise on both sides 3 to 5 times.

Remember to keep your body straight throughout this exercise and to breathe freely.

Form 8. Planting feet solidly on the ground: Stand in a relaxed, at-attention pose. Take a large step to the left so that your feet are wider apart than your shoulders. Raise your arms to shoulder level out to the sides, palms down.

1. Bend your knees and assume a horse-riding or half-squatting posture. Keep your back straight and your head up. At the same time as you are squatting, lower your hands forcefully to a position about 6 inches over your thighs. Your

fingers should be pointing toward each other and naturally spaced, your palms open and facing down. Keep your "tigers' mouths"—the space between your thumbs and forefingers—wide open. (See Fig. 18.)

2. Turn your palms over and slowly but forcefully raise them to chest level as if you were lifting a thousand-pound object. Rise up from your squat at the same slow pace.

Repeat this exercise 3 to 5 times.

Remember that your movements must be slow and steady but forceful. During this exercise make sure that your tongue gently touches the roof of your mouth. Your mouth should be nearly closed but your eyes wide open. Breathe in and out naturally—out while pressing down and in while lifting.

Form 9. Throwing fists from left and right: Stand in the usual starting posture, a relaxed

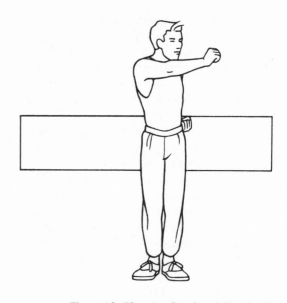

Figure 19. *Throwing fists from left and right*

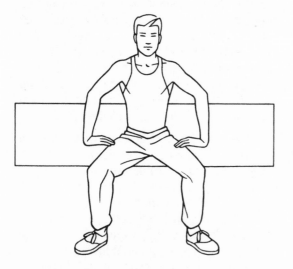

Figure 18. *Planting feet solidly on the ground*

at-attention posture with your feet spaced and your back straight. Bend your elbows back slightly and open your hands with palms up.

1. Turn your hands over and make loose fists. Bend your elbows slightly and draw your fists to the sides of your waist. Then slowly swing your right fist out toward the left, allowing your upper body to turn with the motion. Simultaneously draw your left elbow back. (See Fig. 19.)

2. When you reach the end of the swing, reverse directions. Start withdrawing your right fist back to your side as you begin to swing your left fist out to the right, as in step 1.

Repeat this 3 to 5 times.

Remember that the fist throwing and withdrawing should all be part of one smooth continuous sweep. The withdrawing and extending motions are like waves, steady and uninterrupted. Your breathing should also be coordinated. Breathe in through your nose while swinging your fist out and exhale when it is fully extended.

Form 10. Catching a prey like a fierce tiger: Stand at relaxed attention and let your arms hang down naturally.

1. Take a large step forward with your right foot, bend your right knee and extend your left leg way back far behind you. At the same time, lean forward onto your fingers. You will be in a position similar to a sprinter about to start a race. Keep your head up and your sight fixed ahead. (See Fig. 20.)

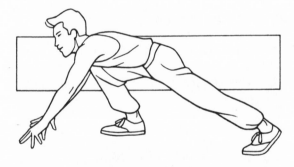

Figure 20. *Catching a prey like a fierce tiger*

2. Bend your arms at the elbows and move your body slightly forward. Move slowly. Imagine that you are a fierce tiger seizing a prey. Then raise your upper body and simultaneously move slightly backward. Repeat this sequence 3 to 5 times. Stand up and bring your right foot back to its original position.

3. Now take one large step forward with your left foot and repeat the sequence in steps 1 and 2.

4. Return to the starting posture. Do this exercise only 1 time with each leg.

Remember that when you are seizing a prey, your waist must be relaxed and your spine concave or flat. Do not arch your back. It is best to touch the ground with all your fingertips. If your fingers are not strong enough to bear your body weight, use your palms instead. Breathe out while moving down and forward. Breathe in while straightening your elbows and moving back. Breathe in through your nose but breathe out through your mouth.

Form 11. Bowing the body: Stand at relaxed attention and let your arms hang down naturally.

1. Wrap your fingers around the back of your head and lace your fingers together. Stretch your elbows to the rear.

2. Bow forward from the waist, keeping your knees straight. Your head is lowered as if you were giving a bow. Keep your knees straight. (See Fig. 21.)

3. In this position, do the exercise called beating heaven's drum. Unlace your hands and place your palms over your ears and your index fingers on top of your middle fingers, then let them slide off to strike your head. Drum 10 to 20 times.

4. Straighten up and let your arms hang naturally.

In the beginning, repeat the bow only 1 or 2 times. Later, you may gradually increase to 3 to 5 times.

Remember not to bend more than you comfortably can. Keep your teeth loosely clenched and your tongue gently touching the roof of your mouth. Breathe lightly or hold your breath until

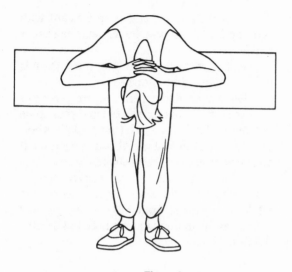

Figure 21. *Bowing the body*

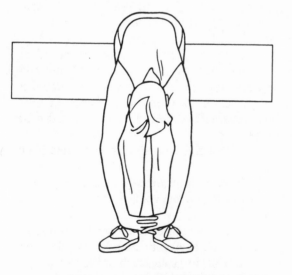

Figure 22. *Wagging the tail*

you straighten up and return to the original position. This exercise is not suitable for patients with high blood pressure or arteriosclerosis.

Form 12. Wagging the tail: Stand in the preparatory posture, loosely at attention with your arms hanging naturally.

1. Raise your hands to the front of your chest and push out with flattened palms until your arms are fully extended.

2. Bring your hands back to your chest, fingers interlocked and palms down.

3. Now lean forward and try to touch the floor with your palms. Keep your legs straight. (See Fig. 22.) Do not force your body to bend, however. Lift your head slightly. Keep your eyes wide open and fix your gaze straight ahead.

4. Straighten up and reach for the sky, rising up on your toes as you do. As you sink down onto the flat of your soles, lower your arms to your sides. Remember to breathe naturally. Patients with high blood pressure or hardening of the arteries in the brain should not do this exercise.

This completes the entire set of *Yee Chin Ching.*

Pa Tuan Chin — The Eight Sets of Embroidery

Pa Tuan Chin, the Eight Sets of Embroidery, is an ancient Chinese exercise, believed to be more than 800 years old. It consists of eight sets of movement. The names of the eight sets are:

1. Holding up the sky with both hands to regulate the *San Chiu* (Triple Warmer) acupuncture meridian.

2. Drawing a bow to the left and to the right as though shooting a bird.

3. Lifting one single hand to regulate the spleen and stomach.

4. Looking backward to get rid of weary and injurious feelings.

5. Wagging head and tail to eliminate the heart's flame.

6. Reaching toes with both hands to strengthen the kidneys and waist.

7. Holding fists and opening angry eyes to increase physical strength.

8. Jolting the back of the body to eliminate disease.

Chin is an embroidered work of silks in various colors. The ancient Chinese broadened the meaning of *chin* to include certain carefully selected and compiled sets of exercise. The eight

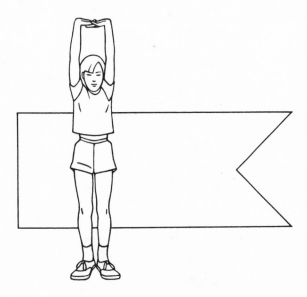

Figure 23. *Holding up the sky with both hands*

sets of specially selected exercise earned the name *Pa Tuan Chin*. The twelve sets of special exercise were called *Shih Erh Tuan Chin.*

Pa Tuan Chin can be performed in either the standing or the bent-knee, horse-riding position. Although it involves moving the trunk, head and neck, its main emphasis is on the arms.

There are two approaches to practicing *Pa Tuan Chin*—movement with force and movement without force. When it is performed with force, the force should be steady, even and potential rather than overt.

Practicing *Pa Tuan Chin* can help you increase your arm and leg strength, develop your chest and prevent improper posture such as saddle or round back. It can help not only the middle-aged and the elderly, but also young people who lack strength or who have improper posture.

Pa Tuan Chin can be practiced with either more force or less force than *Tai Chi Chuan.* The less forceful *Pa Tuan Chin* is more appropriate for the middle-aged and elderly who have average physical strength and for patients with chronic diseases. Here is how to do *Pa Tuan Chin.*

One—Holding up the sky with both hands: Stand at attention with your arms hanging naturally. Look straight ahead.

1. Slowly raise your arms out to the sides, then over your head. With your palms down, lace your fingers together as you lift the heels of your feet approximately 1 inch off the ground.

2. Turn your palms over, keeping your elbows straight. Press up with your hands as you lift your heels further off the ground. (See Fig. 23.) Hold this pose for a few seconds.

3. Release your fingers and slowly bring your arms down sideways, but keep your heels off the ground.

Knocking at the Gate of Life

4. Bring your heels down gently and return to the starting pose.

There is no limit on the number of repetitions. You may do 8 to 16 or as many as you prefer. Do the same number of repetitions for the next seven exercises of *Pa Tuan Chin,* too.

Two—Drawing a bow: Stand in a relaxed state of attention.

1. Take one step to the left and bend your legs to assume a horse-riding posture. Your thighs should be as close as possible to being parallel to the ground. Your back should be straight. Cross your arms in front of your chest with your right arm out and left arm in. Your fingers are loosely separated. Turn your head to the left and look at your right hand.

2. Make a fist with your left hand. Extend both your forefinger and your thumb while keeping the other three fingers curled. Slowly uncurl your left arm to the left until it is fully extended. At the same time, make your right hand into a fist, and draw it to the right as if you were pulling a bow. Your right elbow should be pointing right. Your eyes should be focused on your left forefinger.

3. Relax your left hand and bring it back to the front of your chest at the same time as you are bringing your right hand back. Cross both arms again, this time with your left arm out and your right arm in. Turn to the right and look at your left hand.

4. Make a fist with your right hand. Extend your forefinger and your thumb while keeping the other three fingers curled. Slowly uncurl your right arm to the right until it is fully extended. At the same time, make a fist with your left hand and draw your left elbow to the left as though pulling a bow. Your eyes should stay on your right forefinger. (See Fig. 24.)

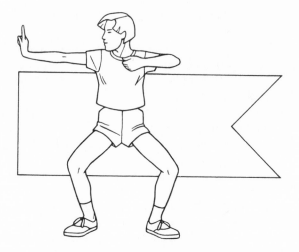

Figure 24. *Drawing a bow*

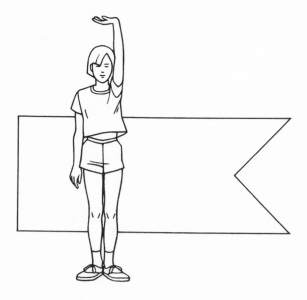

Figure 25. *Lifting one single hand*

Three—Lifting one single hand: Stand loosely at attention with your arms hanging naturally.

1. Flex your left hand back toward the wrist, keeping your fingers together and your elbow straight. Raise that arm out to the left and then over your head. Your palms should be up and your fingers pointing right. At the same time, stretch your right hand down toward the floor, your palm facing back. (See Fig. 25.)

2. Bring your left hand down in a slow semicircle to the left, and stretch it toward the floor with your palm facing back. At the same time, flex your right hand back toward your wrist and raise it in a slow semicircle to the right until it is over your head. Your fingers are together, your arm is fully extended, your palm is up and your fingers are pointing left.

Four—Looking backward: Stand at relaxed attention. Hold your head up straight. Let your arms hang naturally, but press your palms tightly against your outer thighs.

1. Keep your chest upright and pull your shoulders slightly back. At the same time, turn your head slowly to the left and look behind you.

2. Relax your head and shoulders, turn to the front and look straight ahead.

3. Keep your chest upright and pull your shoulders slightly back. At the same time, turn your head slowly to the right, and look behind you. (See Fig. 26.)

4. Bring your head and shoulders back to the starting position and look straight ahead.

Five—Wagging head and tail: Separate your feet to a distance equal to about 3 times the length of one of your feet. Bend your knees and assume a horse-riding posture. Place your hands

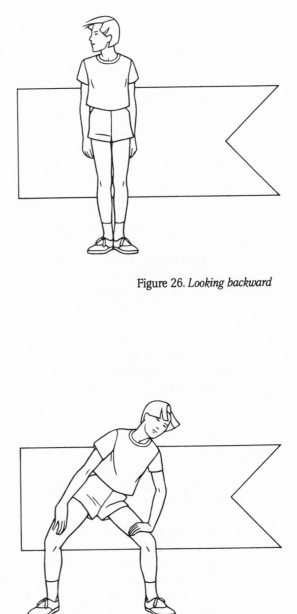

Figure 26. *Looking backward*

Figure 27. *Wagging head and tail*

just above your knees with your "tigers' mouths" —the space between your thumbs and forefingers—facing in toward your body. Keep your upper body straight.

1. Bend your upper body low to the left front with your head down. (See Fig. 27.) Swing your head and upper body in a clockwise circle in front of you. You'll find that as your head circles, your buttocks will make a smaller circle in the opposite direction. This is head and tail wagging.

2. Stop the circle when you are leaning right, and return to the starting position— squatting as if riding a horse but with your back straight.

3. Bend your upper body low to the right front and circle counterclockwise. Stop circling, but remain in the horse-riding posture for a moment or two.

Six—Reaching toes with both hands: Stand in a relaxed at-attention posture.

1. Bend your upper body slowly forward with your knees straight and touch your toes or ankles. Keep your head very slightly raised. (See Fig. 28a.)

2. Straighten up and return to the preparatory posture.

3. Place your hands in the small of your back. Slowly bend backward. (See Fig. 28b.)

4. Return to the preparatory posture.

Seven—Holding fists and opening angry eyes: Space your feet more than a shoulder width apart. Bend your knees and assume a horse-riding posture. Place your fists at the sides of your waist, fingers facing up.

1. Extend your left arm slowly forward until your fist is straight out in front of you, fingers facing down. At the same time, clench

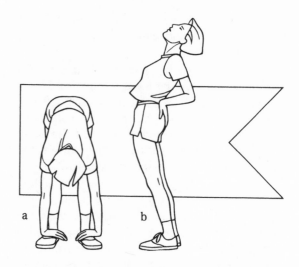

a   b

Figure 28. *Reaching toes with both hands*

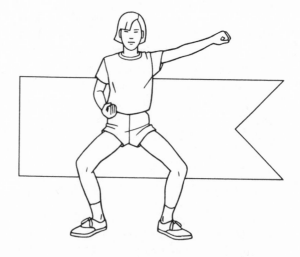

Figure 29. *Holding fists and opening angry eyes*

your right fist tightly and pull your elbow to the rear. Open your eyes wide and glare at objects in front of you. (See Fig. 29.)

2. Draw both fists back to the sides of your waist. Repeat the exercise, reversing the position of your arms.

3. Return to the starting position with your fists at your sides.

Eight—Jolting the back: Stand at attention. Keep your toes together, with your palms flat against your thighs.

1. Stand up very straight. Propel your head straight up by lifting your heels high off the ground. (See Fig. 30.)

2. Lower your heels and stand in the starting position.

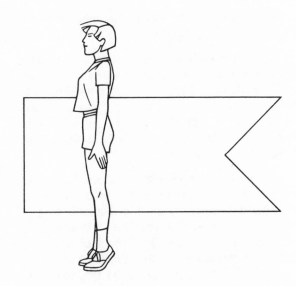

Figure 30. *Jolting the back*

Shih Erh Tuan Chin—The Twelve Sets of Embroidery

Shih Erh Tuan Chin, The Twelve Sets of Embroidery, is a remarkably effective exercise that has been popular with the common people in China for many centuries.

Shih Erh Tuan Chin consists of self-massage and fitness exercises. The first eleven exercises can be performed in a cross-legged position or in a regular sitting position. (The twelfth exercise is done in a standing position.) And they can be done even by the old and weak or those suffering from chronic diseases.

Both testimony from the past and modern observation make it clear that this exercise has preventive and therapeutic value.

Here are the embroidery exercises and the benefits you will get from them.

One—Teeth tapping: Tap your upper and lower teeth against each other 20 to 30 times. This exercise helps stimulate the blood vessels in your gums. It improves the circulation in the area and strengthens your teeth. It helps prevent dental diseases. But if you have serious gum disease or uneven teeth, you should not do this exercise.

Two—Tongue revolving: Move the tip of your tongue against your teeth in all directions —back and forth, left and right, up and down. Do it until your mouth feels tingly. This exercise has a massaging effect on the gums, and the mucous membrane of the mouth cavity. It contributes to a successful treatment of bleeding and receding gums. It also keeps the mouth

30

Knocking at the Gate of Life

cavity clean, stimulates the secretion of saliva and speeds up digestion.

Three—Face rubbing: First rub your palms rapidly against each other to create some warmth. Then lightly rub your face with your palms 20 to 30 times. This action can help improve blood circulation in the skin and help maintain elasticity. However, persons with boils should not perform this exercise.

Four—Beating heaven's drum: First cover your ears with the base of your palms and place your forefingers on top of your middle fingers. Then let your forefingers slide off your middle fingers so that they strike the back of your head in the vicinity of the acupuncture point *Feng Chih*—Windy Lake. (See Fig. 31.) Do this 20 to 30 times. You will hear a drumlike sound.

This action can relieve dizziness and headache. According to traditional Chinese medical theory, the *Feng Chih* point is part of the Foot-Gallbladder-Lesser Yang meridian. Applying acupuncture techniques to this particular point can treat headache, dizziness and stiffness of the neck and collarbone area. Striking the *Feng Chih* point with the forefinger is in essence massaging this point with the point-rapping technique. This exercise can not only relieve symptoms but can also prevent them from happening.

Five—Wheel-turning: Make your hands into fists over your head with your knuckles pointing forward. Bend your elbows slightly and bring your arms forward and back as if you were spinning a water wheel. Do this 10 or more times. This exercise is effective in preventing arthritic changes in the shoulder joints.

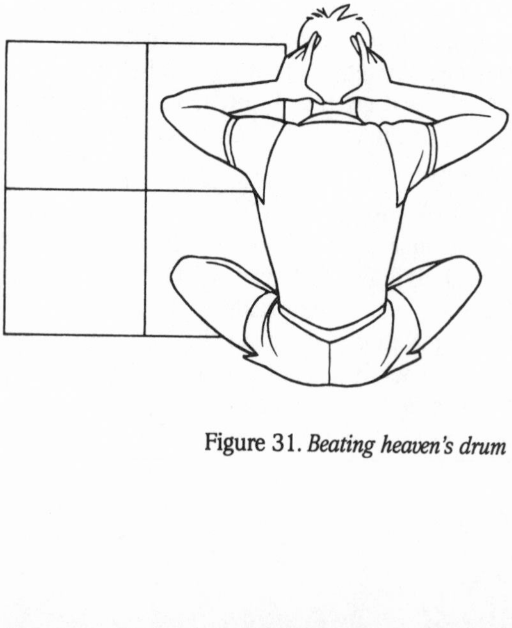

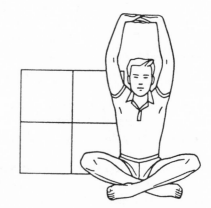

Figure 32. *Holding up the sky*

Figure 31. *Beating heaven's drum*

Six—Holding up the sky: Clasp your hands with your fingers interlocked in front of you. Turn your palms over and stretch your arms above your head as if you were holding up the sky. (See Fig. 32.) Do this 10 or more times. This exercise can expand your chest and facilitate deep breathing.

Seven—Drawing a bow in two directions: Mimic the motions of drawing and shooting a bow. (See Fig. 33.) Alternate hands and sides. Do this 10 or more times. This exercise also stretches and expands your chest. In addition, it trains your shoulder joints and adds strength to your arms.

Eight—Lowering the head and touching the toes: Sit on the floor with your legs fully extended. Lean forward and touch your toes with your hands. (See Fig. 34.) Do this 10 or more times.

Since this exercise involves moving the waist and abdomen, it is relatively demanding. It stretches the muscles in your waist, back and thighs. It also contributes to flexibility in the spine and to the overall health of your body.

Nine—Rubbing *Tan Tien:* *Tan Tien* is generally believed to be located 1.5 to 2 *ts'uns* (Chinese inches) below the navel—that's about

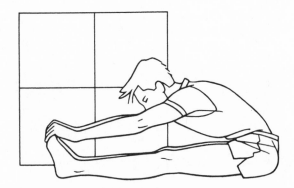

Figure 34. *Lowering the head and touching the toes*

3 Western inches. Rubbing *Tan Tien* is in essence rubbing your lower abdomen. Rub this area with three fingers of your right hand for 30 or more rotations. *Tan Tien* is very near the *Shih Men* (Stone Gate) point, which is found about 2 *ts'uns* below the navel. According to Chinese medical theory, *Shih Men* belongs to *Jen Mo*, The Conception Vessel, an acupuncture meridian. Applying stimulation to this point can relieve indigestion, abdominal pain and nocturnal emission. You may well notice a lessening of these symptoms after massaging this point.

Ten—Rubbing *Shen Yu* **(Respectable Kidney):** Rub your hands briskly against each other to create warmth. Then place your palms against the back of your waist, as in Fig. 35, to massage the *Shen Yu* (Respectable Kidney) points located here. Rub at least 20 to 30 times. This exercise is very helpful in preventing lower back pain and improving your health in general.

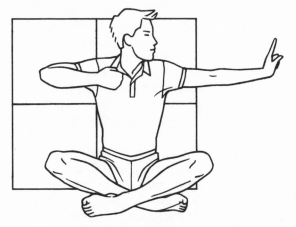

Figure 33. *Drawing a bow in two directions*

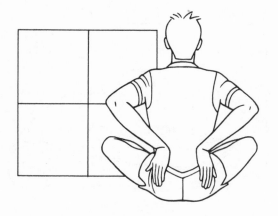

Figure 35. *Rubbing* Shen Yu *(Respectable Kidney)*

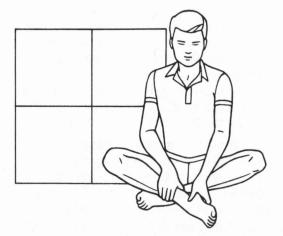

Figure 36. *Rubbing* Yung Chuan *(Bubbling Spring)*

Eleven—Rubbing *Yung Chuan* **(Bubbling Spring):** First rub your hands against each other to create warmth. Then rub the sole of your left foot with the three middle fingers of your right hand until heat is generated. Next rub the sole of your right foot with your left hand in the same manner. (See Fig. 36.)

According to traditional Chinese medical theory, *Yung Chuan,* which is located in the middle of the sole of the foot, is the starting point of the Foot-Lesser Yin-Kidney meridian. Massaging this point can cause what is called "insubstantial heat" to descend. This assists in the treatment of insomnia and heart palpitations. It also can improve your walking.

Twelve—Foot treading: You do this exercise standing up. Plant one foot at a time firmly on the ground, one after the other. Do this 10 or more times. This exercise can revitalize blood circulation as well as stretch the muscles and supportive tissues of the leg.

These exercises can be performed after getting up in the morning or before bedtime. They can be performed in whole or in part, depending on your condition. The order of the exercises and the number of repetitions may also be varied to meet your individual needs and convenience. For instance, someone suffering from a strained groin muscle might rub *Shen Yu* several hundred times in a row with good results. Of course, most people will find rubbing 30 times sufficient.

The therapeutic and preventive values of *Shih Erh Tuan Chin* and other similar exercises have been well documented throughout their long history. You should expect a significant improvement in your health if you persistently perform these exercises over weeks and months.

The Chinese and Waist Training

Chinese exercises are guided by traditional Chinese medical theory. According to the *Ching Lo* theory, which deals with pathways of *ch'i*—energy—the exact center of the back of the waist is the pathway of the *Tu Mo,* or Governor Vessel. *Tu Mo,* which is related to the kidneys, runs through the spine. When *Tu Mo* is free from obstruction, *shen ch'i,* kidney *ch'i* or energy, will be in abundant supply.

In addition, the acupuncture point *Shen Yu,* Respectable Kidney, which is located at the side of the waist, is also closely related to the condition of *shen ch'i,* kidney energy. Thus, exercising the waist area regularly will enable *ch'i* to circulate freely in the *Tu Mo* and will also stimulate the *Shen Yu* point. As a result, the kidneys will be full of energy. Since the kidneys store *ching*—the fundamental substance—it follows that when the kidneys have an abundant supply of energy, then *ching ch'i,* the essential energy of life, will also be richly available. And *yuan ch'i,* the primary vital energy, will be vigorous in the maintenance of health. For this reason, the traditional Chinese fitness exercises pay special attention to the training of the waist region. For example, waist training is considered to be the focal point in *Tai Chi Chuan.* Movements involving the waist can also be found in *Pa Tuan Chin* and *Yee Chin Ching.*

From the standpoint of modern physiology and anatomy, frequent exercise of the waist can keep the spine flexible and facilitate blood circulation in the abdominal and pelvic cavities. The result is the same whatever the theory—an improvement in health.

In addition to *Tai Chi Chuan* and *Pa Tuan Chin,* there are some additional traditional Chinese exercises that stress the movement of the waist.

Body bending: After getting up in the morning, bend at the waist to lower your upper body. Stretch the waist, then stand up. Do this 20 to 100 times. Your movements may be either swift or slow.

Bean picking: Place a number of beans, wooden blocks or any small object on the floor. With your knees straight, bend at the waist to pick up the blocks or beans. After picking up one or two, stand up slowly. Repeat this movement until you have picked up all the beans.

Rowing a long oar with both hands: Stand with one foot forward and one foot a step behind. Hold your hands out in front of you as if you were grasping a long oar. Push your hands forward and down and bend your upper body and head to the front. Then draw your hands and upper body back and up to your original position. As you do this exercise, you may take one step forward with each sweep of the "oar" if you wish. The sweep of your rowing may also be increased gradually.

Turning the body to look behind: Stand with your feet apart and your arms slightly bent, palms down. Swing your upper body from side to side. As you turn in each direction, you should be able to see your heels.

The Benefits of *Tai Chi Chuan*

"*Tai Chi Chuan* is good medicine for chronic disease." "*Tai Chi Chuan* is a valuable fitness exercise for the elderly." Remarks such as these are based on a solid foundation. Centuries of successful use of *Tai Chi Chuan* testify to the health-improving benefits of this gentle flowing system known as the Supreme Ultimate Exercise.

To know *Tai Chi* fully, you should study with someone who has already mastered this art. Involved is the memorization over a period of time of a graceful dancelike routine and the progressive learning of the proper attitude of relaxation. But if there are no *Tai Chi* classes available to you or if you prefer to work alone, you may still get most of the benefits of this splendid exercise. The illustrations on pages 37 to 39 show the first set of the *Tai Chi* routine. Along with the description of *Tai Chi* starting on page 36, they can help you understand the form and movement of this exercise.

In fact, it is not necessary to follow the exact motion of *Tai Chi* to get good results. On the opposing page, there is a section on doing *Tai Chi*-type movements. It must be noted in all honesty, however, that *Tai Chi* is so unique that if you possibly can, you should arrange to see it actually done at least once.

Doing *Tai Chi* will benefit your cardiovascular system, first of all. It will help prevent high blood pressure and arteriosclerosis. According to one survey, the average blood pressure of elderly persons who regularly practiced *Tai Chi Chuan* was 134/80 as compared to an average reading of 154/82 for those who didn't. The *Tai Chi* group also had a lower incidence of hardening of the blood vessels by 38 percent to 46 percent. Moreover, the cardiovascular functioning of all subjects in the *Tai Chi* group was normal. But 35 percent of the other group had inadequate cardiac function. There's just no doubt that regular practice of *Tai Chi Chuan* can benefit the cardiovascular system.

Second, *Tai Chi* helps keep your bones and joints in good condition, preventing problems in those areas. According to one report, elderly *Tai Chi* practitioners had only 26 percent age-induced spinal changes compared to 47 percent in the control group. They also enjoyed better spinal mobility than their non-exercising counterparts. A great majority of the *Tai Chi* group—more than 85 percent, in fact—were able to reach the ground with their fingertips without bending their knees. But only 21 percent of the control group could do so. Further, the *Tai Chi* group had few problems with brittle bones.

Practicing *Tai Chi* helps the body maintain overall good health and prevents *shun shi*—kidney deficiency. According to traditional Chinese medical theory, *shun shi* signals deterioration or weakness in the overall functioning of the body. Most elderly *Tai Chi* exercisers studied did not show *shun shi,* but half of those who were inactive did.

Tai Chi Chuan has additional benefits for the nervous system, digestion, respiratory system, bones, joints and muscles. *Tai Chi* regularly practiced can, indeed, improve physical fitness and prevent disease.

Why *Tai Chi* Is Special

Tai Chi Chuan is a Chinese exercise of physical fitness that has a long tradition. An extraction of the very best elements from a variety of ancient Chinese exercises, *Tai Chi Chuan* has for many centuries remained popular with the common people. In recent years, *Tai Chi Chuan* has attracted worldwide attention both in the medical and sport arenas. It has crossed national boundaries and become one of the most important and popular international therapeutic exercises.

The fact that *Tai Chi Chuan* has become popular is not accidental at all. It consists of movements that are so soft, steady, smooth and slow that it is suitable for everybody, even the elderly and the physically weak. It requires relaxation of the muscles of the wrist, arms, shoulders, chest, abdomen and back. The softness of its movements and its required muscular relaxation contribute to a peaceful and refreshed feeling. The cerebral cortex becomes calm and rested. In this way, practicing *Tai Chi* can relieve neurosis and depression.

The muscular relaxation also conditions the blood vessels to dilate, which lowers blood pressure. Practicing *Tai Chi* is, therefore, an effective treatment for high blood pressure.

Tai Chi is calming. It's guided by *yi*—concentration—and by peaceful passive focusing, rather than by force. By producing a proper balance between sympathetic excitation and inhibition, *Tai Chi* effectively treats both anxiety and depression.

And *Tai Chi* involves the whole body. Each movement strengthens and tones a different group of muscles and joints. Consistent practice makes joints more flexible and ligaments more elastic. It also increases muscular strength.

Tai Chi breathing must be deep but quiet, long but rhythmic. Because the breathing and movements especially stimulate the waist region, blood circulation in the abdomen is enhanced and stomach and intestinal movement is speeded up.

Since the exertion required by *Tai Chi* can be adjusted to suit individual needs, everyone—male or female, old or young, the fit or the weak—can do this exercise. The physically weak, for example, can practice the high form—the one that doesn't require squatting down low. Or they can do the simplified version instead of the whole set. And, of course, the physically strong can do the low form which requires strength to maintain a bent-legged position.

Generally speaking, *Tai Chi Chuan* imposes little physiological demand on the body. After completing a whole set of the simplified version, for example, the average pulse rate of a group of adolescent students was only 105 and their blood pressure 128/70. Three minutes after finishing the set, both the pulse rate and the blood pressure of these youngsters had returned to the pre-exercise level. During the exercise, their breathing was not even hard, and in one 5-minute session, only about 12 calories were consumed. Because it's so physically undemanding, *Tai Chi* is ideally suited to the elderly, the physically weak and chronic disease patients.

Tai Chi can help everyone develop grace, coordination and balance. The flowing, intricate and orderly steps demand these qualities. Forms such as "brushing knee and twist step," "turning over the arm," and "waving hands like clouds" develop coordination. "Left and right foot separation" and "stand with one foot bent," for instance, teach balance.

The Way of *Tai Chi Chuan*

To get the best results and the maximum benefits from *Tai Chi,* you need a vision of how the exercise should be practiced.

First, see yourself moving your body softly and breathing in and out naturally. The movements of *Tai Chi Chuan* must be continuous, soft, slow, gentle, measured and smooth. You must try to walk like a cat and move like silk off the reel.

The whole set of simplified *Tai Chi Chuan* usually takes 4 to 6 minutes. It's perfectly okay, however, to take as long as 8 or 9 minutes and perform it in slow motion.

Beginners should breathe naturally. You shouldn't breathe hard, pant or hold your breath. After you have become proficient, you may coordinate movements with your breathing. You may, for example, breathe in as you move up and breathe out as you move down. Or breathe in as you move in and breathe out as you move out. Breathe with your abdomen, deeply and naturally.

Second, keep your body loose and comfortable. Maintain a balance between activity and placidness. Artificial force and unnatural strength should not be applied in performing *Tai Chi.* You should, instead, relax your entire body and keep your posture natural and comfortable. It is especially important to relax the waist, abdomen and chest muscles. Do not hold your chest out stiffly.

Let your back muscles stretch out and be comfortable. Let your shoulders be loose and hang naturally. Allow your elbows to relax. In China, this stance is called *han hsiung pa pei*—the chest-embracing, back-expanding pose, and *chen ch'ien chai chou*—the loose-shoulders, relaxed-elbows posture. This posture will enable you to feel natural and comfortable, and to maintain a stable center of gravity.

While doing *Tai Chi,* you must be mentally quiet and peaceful. Concentrate fully on the movements and avoid distractions.

The goal is to integrate *hsing*—physical form—with *yi*—concentration. You want to internalize force and strength.

Hsing refers to the body's movement, and *yi* refers to consciousness. Integrating *hsing* and *yi* in *Tai Chi* means that you aim to guide and control your body movements with your thought. You should visualize the form as you do it. Then

there is perfect agreement between what you are thinking and what you are doing.

In *Tai Chi Chuan,* the force and power must be internally restrained and should not be externally revealed. The muscles should never be tensed to create force and power.

Exercise from *Tai Chi*

People who have not successfully learned the whole *Tai Chi Chuan* routine for one reason or another may practice *Tai Chi* movement exercises instead. In essence, this is a freestyle exercise that you invent as you go along, based very loosely on the grace, fluidity, slowness and softness of *Tai Chi.*

The requirement of *Tai Chi* movement exercises are the same as those for *Tai Chi Chuan,* described on page 35. Briefly, the requirements are to relax your entire body. You can do this by practicing exercise 14 on page 85. Those who cannot practice this exercise because of poor health may skip it and proceed directly to the *Tai Chi* movement exercises.

The next requirement is that you breathe naturally. After relaxing your body, make sure to relax your respiratory muscles as well. The speed and frequency of your breathing should be allowed to follow their natural courses. Breathe in and out through your nose, or with both your nose and mouth.

Third, concentrate mentally. To reduce distractions, you may leave your eyes partially closed or fully opened, whichever is most relaxing. Gently focus your attention on the area of your navel.

Move softly. After your body is completely relaxed, you can start to make movements. Keep your knees slightly bent at all times when your body is in motion. You may move your body any

(continued on page 40)

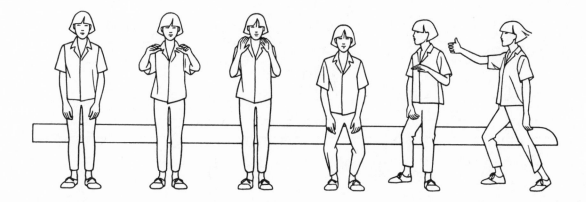

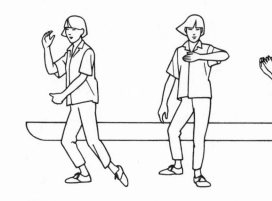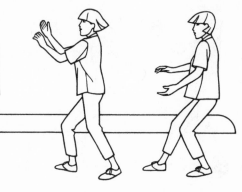

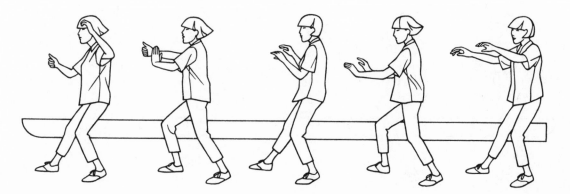

Figure 37. *The first set of* Tai Chi

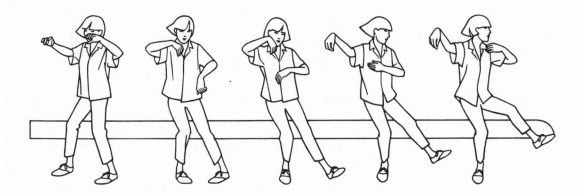

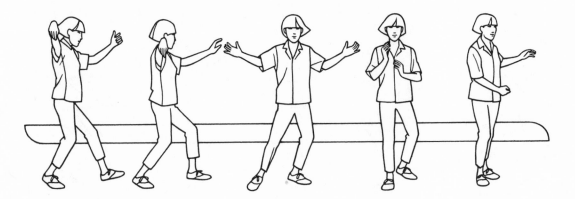

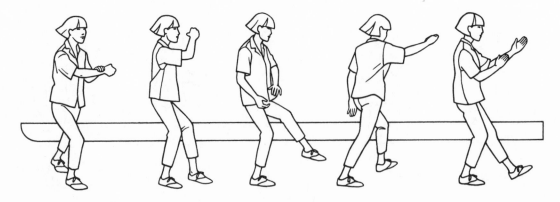

Figure 37. *The first set of* Tai Chi

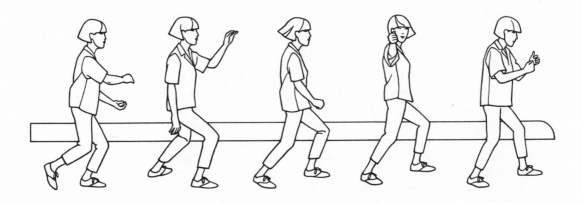

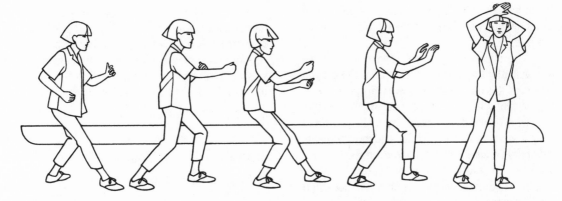

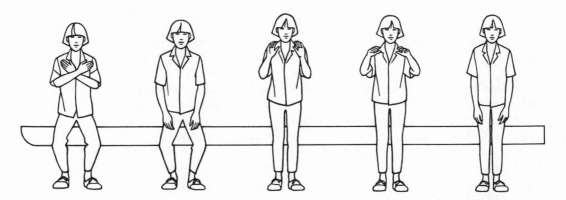

Figure 37. *The first set of* Tai Chi

way you want in any approximate imitation of the movements of *Tai Chi Chuan.*

Let your trunk, your arms and your legs move freely without the slightest restraint. After practicing for a period of time, you will be able to move softly and slowly. You may find that your hands and feet have become more graceful. The movement will become increasingly spontaneous. Do not be concerned about performing any special movements nor deliberately seek after them. Let them come naturally.

When you want to terminate the exercise, you should do so slowly. After stopping, walk for a few minutes and breathe deeply a few times. Or you may like to massage your head for a while.

The effects of *Tai Chi* movement exercise are basically the same as those of *Tai Chi Chuan.* However, it is much easier to learn and to do, and consequently, has a greater appeal to more people.

In order to do this exercise well, you must fully understand the principles and requirements of *Tai Chi Chuan.* In addition to becoming familiar with the sections in this book dealing with *Tai Chi,* you should also read some other books on the Supreme Ultimate Exercise.

Why Chinese Massage Is Unique

The Chinese health protection massage was classified as *Dao Yin*—gymnastic exercise—in ancient China. Designed to maintain and improve health, it is a self-massage.

Chinese massage, called *An Mu,* differs from Western self-massage in a number of ways. Based on the Chinese medical theory *Ching Lo,* which concerns the pathways of *ch'i* or energy, Chinese massage places special emphasis on acupuncture points such as *Yung Chuan* (Bubbling Spring), *Shen Yu* (Respectable Kidney), *Tan Tien* (Cinnabar Field) and *Yin Shen* (Welcome Fragrance). On the other hand, the Western type focuses on massaging the muscles.

An Mu pays special attention to massaging the head and waist regions. The Western type emphasizes massaging the limbs.

An Mu typically uses the techniques of knocking, beating and patting. It is common in Chinese massage, for example, to knock against the shoulders and abdomen, to pat the legs with palm or fist, and to beat around the waist with palm or fist. On the other hand, Western massage relies mainly on kneading and rubbing and puts much less emphasis on knocking, beating or patting.

Mental concentration, relaxation and calmness are required in the application of Chinese massage. There are no such requirements in Western massage.

How *Ch'i Kung* Builds Energy and Health

Ch'i Kung is a *kung fu*—mastery of a mental or physical feat through systematic practice. It is designed to train or condition *ch'i,* energy. A unique Chinese fitness method, *Ch'i Kung* is an effective technique for preventing disease.

In Chinese medical theory, *ch'i* refers both to the air one inhales and *yuen ch'i*—the primary vital energy stored in the body. To condition *ch'i* is, in essence, to condition *yuen ch'i. Yuen ch'i* may be considered as being roughly equivalent to the sum total of the body's ability to resist disease, to adapt to the external environment and to restore proper internal functioning.

Traditional Chinese medicine recognizes that an abundant supply of *yuen ch'i* is vital to maintaining health and preventing disease. According to these theories, when *cheng ch'i,* the inherent energy, is internally stored and *yuen ch'i* is abundantly available, there will be no room for a disease to invade. For this reason, Chinese medicine pays particular attention to cultivating *yuen ch'i* as a means of preventing disease. When a disease does occur, it is important to restore *yuen ch'i* through various means to speed up recovery. *Ch'i Kung* conditions and nourishes this vital energy to improve physical stamina and health.

In general, *Ch'i Kung* consists of three parts. It adjusts your body posture. It adjusts your respiration or breathing cycle. And it adjusts your mind and nervous system. These three components are interdependent. Each one affects the other two. To learn the techniques of *Ch'i Kung,* you must understand and develop all three fundamental principles.

There are various types of *Ch'i Kung.* The most popular types today, however, are *Fang Sung Kung,* which is relaxation breathing; *Ch'iang Chuang Kung,* invigorative breathing, and *Nei Yang Kung,* or internally nourishing breathing.

How *Ch'i Kung* Relieves Disease

For healing, *Ch'i Kung* is mainly used against chronic diseases. Clinical evidence collected in China in recent years indicates that *Ch'i Kung* is relatively effective in treating depression and anxiety, high blood pressure, gastric and duodenal ulcers, other stomach troubles and habitual constipation. For other chronic diseases, *Ch'i Kung* contributes to the treatment process through improving the body's overall health.

Ch'i Kung is effective in treating disease because it nourishes *yuen ch'i,* your primary vital

energy, through mental quietness. Nourishing *yuen ch'i* restores vital energy that has been consumed, gradually increases the body's resistance to disease and systematically restores impaired body functions.

According to studies of the brain, the state of mental quietness known as *ju ching* in *Ch'i Kung* corresponds to a state in which cortical or thinking brain activities are internally inhibited. Under the protection of such internal inhibition, the overstimulated and overworked nerve cells in the cortex can be rejuvenated, and the excitability of the cortex can be neutralized.

Such an internal condition provides a favorable condition for physical recuperation. That *Ch'i Kung* is effective in treating depression, anxiety, ulcers and high blood pressure may be attributed to its beneficial effects on the nervous system. The development of these diseases is closely related to the condition of the individual's nervous system and mental state.

Scientific research has also verified that *Ch'i Kung* contributes to the process both of sparing energy and of accumulating reserves of energy. In some ways, these changes are measurable. During the practice of *Ch'i Kung,* for instance, oxygen consumption is reduced by 31 percent, and the metabolic rate by about 20 percent.

This energy-saving reaction helps you get greater mileage from a smaller output of energy and helps to restore your depleted energy reserves. The reason *Ch'i Kung* is effective in treating chronic disease of the "fiery" type as well as in restoring the energy level of the physically weak is probably related to *Ch'i Kung's* ability to save energy.

The breathing movement of *Ch'i Kung* effectively massages the organs inside the abdominal cavity perhaps even more thoroughly than if you used your hands. The massage from abdominal breathing, a typical breathing style of the *Nei Yang Kung*, or internally nourishing style, is especially vigorous.

During *Chi'i Kung* the diaphragm may move three to four times as far as it does in ordinary breathing. In doing so, it massages organs within the abdominal cavity. This can speed up stomach and intestinal movement, reduce abdominal sluggishness and improve digestion and absorption. That is why weak and underweight exercisers, after practicing *Ch'i Kung*, will usually feel an increase in their appetites, consume more food and add pounds to their body weight. Because of its massaging action, *Ch'i Kung* can be especially effective against both a general rundown condition and habitual constipation.

Becoming a *Ch'i Kung* Master

To fully master the techniques of *Ch'i Kung*, you must adhere to several principles. First of all, you must be relaxed and natural. When practicing *Ch'i Kung*, you must allow both your body and your mind to get loose.

To relax your body, you should loosen your belt and your clothes. You must not raise your shoulders nor elevate your chest. You shouldn't try too hard to hold your body posture in an unnatural pose. If you don't feel comfortable with a posture, you should adjust yourself so that you are free from any constraints. Most important, you must relax your muscles, particularly the muscles of your lower abdomen.

The second requirement is that you must relax your mind. It will help if you put a happy expression on your face. Become composed. During the exercise, you must concentrate and avoid the slightest distraction.

After you have achieved this initial relaxation, you should pay attention to regulating your breathing rhythm. The manner in which you exhale can frequently indicate whether or not both body and mind are in a state of relaxation.

To achieve mental quietness while engaging in *Ch'i Kung*, you must focus your thought and consciousness completely on the exercise itself. By doing so, you will be able to keep distracting thoughts and diversions by such things as sound and light to the minimum. It is not unusual for a *Ch'i Kung* exerciser to temporarily lose the sensation of body weight upon entering into a state of mental serenity.

Of course, it is normal for beginners to be diverted from concentration by distractions. If this occurs, you may mentally suggest to yourself that you need to be patient and that you have the will to overcome this problem. Such mental suggestions will often calm the mind. With persistent practice, your mental concentration will gradually improve.

In practicing *Ch'i Kung*, you must integrate the training of *yi*, your consciousness, with the training of *ch'i*, regulating your respiration. You must learn how to direct the movement of *ch'i* with your consciousness. In other words, let your thought control your breathing. Allow your consciousness to adjust the regularity, duration, volume and speed of your breathing. Through conditioning, you will ultimately be able to lead or follow the movement of *ch'i* with *yi*.

To condition *yi* is to attain mental quietness. To condition *ch'i* is to regulate your breathing by following the implications of these seven words —*narrow, deep, long, slow, steady, soft* and *even*. While *Ch'iang Chuang Kung* and *Fang Sung Kung*, the relaxation and the invigorating techniques, place greater emphasis on conditioning *yi, Nei Yang Kung*, the internally nourishing method, focuses more on conditioning *ch'i*. Whatever the method used, all techniques of *Ch'i Kung* are designed to integrate *yi* with *ch'i*.

Ch'i Kung attempts to achieve a state of mental tranquility and quietness without involving the movement of the body. In order to maintain a proper balance between body movement and mental quietness, you should also engage in other forms of therapeutic exercises. Better therapeutic effects can be achieved when combining *Ch'i Kung* with action-oriented exercises. *Ch'i Kung*, however, should be performed before the other exercises.

Ch'i Kung Step by Step

As a *kung fu, Ch'i Kung* must be practiced regularly, following a gradual process, to reach proficiency. It cannot be done overnight.

To develop the proper body posture and to master the breathing techniques, you must begin with the easy ones before attempting to do the more complicated ones. You must also follow the procedure step by step to learn the technique of *ju ching*—entering into a state of mental quietness. In the beginning, your practice session should be brief, no more than 15 or 20 minutes. Later, it may be longer.

About 10 or 15 minutes before engaging in the exercise, you should terminate all mental work and eliminate body wastes.

Set the amount of time for the exercise based on your health, fitness and mood. After the exercise is over, don't stand up immediately. First rub your face with both hands and gently massage your eyes before getting up slowly. Stretch both your arms and legs.

If during the exercise you find your breathing rhythm shallow and uneven, you should look for the cause of the problem. It's very likely that it's caused either by an incorrect method of breathing, an unpleasant frame of mind, lack of desire to do the exercise or mental distractions. Correct the problem before continuing.

If you get a headache, dizziness or a sensation of heaviness in your head, your problem most likely results from trying so hard that you cause an unnatural breathing rhythm. Impatience and emotional agitation may be responsible. Find the cause and correct it.

Don't do *Ch'i Kung* either right after a meal or on an empty stomach. Nor should you practice *Ch'i Kung* when you have a fever, diarrhea, a bad cold or are simply physically tired.

Strange Sensations and *Ch'i Kung*

When properly done, you will not normally have any unusual reactions from practicing *Fang Sung Kung, Ch'iang Chuang Kung* and *Nei Yang Kung*. It is not unusual, however, for beginners occasionally to experience certain out-of-the-ordinary reactions because they have not yet become accustomed to the new posture, breathing rhythm and the requirements for mental concentration. Failure to practice the exercise correctly may also lead to problems. In general, abnormal reactions can be prevented or overcome by making necessary adjustments. Following are some possible problems and ways to handle them.

Postural problems: If you have soreness and pain in your waist and back, the cause is most often the use of an uncomfortable or inappropriate sitting position. You can overcome this by starting the exercise in the lying-down position before working up to the sitting position. Or whenever you feel tired, you may immediately switch to the lying-down position. Another alternative is simply to reduce the sitting time.

If your feet get numb when you sit cross-legged, you may do some leg bending and stretching exercises before you sit down. If you still get numbness, you can massage your feet or switch the position of the foot that is on top. You may also get up and do something else for a while before sitting down again.

Breathing problems: If you have an unsteady breathing rhythm or uncomfortable feelings connected with your respiration, it's probably due to the beginner's failure to follow the correct breathing procedure because of impatience. Instead of letting your breathing occur naturally, you may have attempted to force your breathing to become deep and long. This problem can be corrected simply by allowing your breathing to become spontaneous and natural. If you want, you can walk around indoors for a while to allow your emotions to calm down before returning to the exercise.

Some beginners experience congestion and a feeling of obstruction in their chests and pain around their ribs. This problem is most often caused by breathing with too much force or by holding your breath for too long. These reactions may also occur if you stop inhaling at the chest or throat level. You can avoid these abnormal reactions by using the correct method for breathing.

Problems with mental concentration: Drowsiness and sleepiness can occur when the exerciser who is very tired practices *Ch'i Kung* in the lying-down position. To overcome it, you can switch to a sitting position. Or you can open your eyes slightly and look at your nose tip.

As a rule, it is not desirable to practice *Ch'i Kung* when you are tired. It is quite natural, however, for the beginner sometimes to fall asleep. To prevent drowsiness, you may find it helpful to drink a little hot tea and walk a few steps indoors before engaging in *Ch'i Kung*.

Sometimes after entering into a state of mental quietness, you may find that a part of your skin has begun itching or burning, feels like insects are crawling on it or just feels numb. These are most often illusions. Do not pay special attention to them. They will go away if you continue to focus your attention on the lower abdomen, and if you avoid overly deep or long breathing.

Other symptoms: Occasionally people experience palpitations after entering into the state of quietness. Most often they are caused by a too lengthy inhalation or holding the breath for too long, but they may also result from emotional agitation. Correct the problem by maintaining a smooth breathing rhythm and calming your emotions.

If you get a throbbing sensation in your temporal artery when doing *Ch'i Kung* while lying on your side, you can eliminate it by changing the position of your head to take pressure off your ear.

Fang Sung Kung— Relaxation Breathing

Fang Sung Kung, the relaxation breathing exercise, can be used to help treat all kinds of chronic diseases. It is relatively easy to do.

To begin, take a supine position as shown in Fig. 38. Lie upon a thick pillow and support your shoulders and back with a towel or sheeting. Keep your head straight and your arms extended beside your body. Your legs should be stretched out naturally. Keep your eyes partially closed. Close your mouth naturally and let your upper and lower teeth gently touch each other. The tip of your tongue will be slightly against the roof of your mouth.

Breathe naturally in and out through your nose. The rhythm and depth of your breathing are basically the same as normal everyday breathing. What is important is that you regulate your breathing so that it's narrow, which means it should be soundless; smooth, which means it has an even speed and depth; and steady, which means it should be unrestrained and unobstructed.

The method of *ju ching*, entering into quietness, involves using certain words to induce relaxation. While you are inhaling, think of the word *quiet*. As you exhale, think of the word *relax*. While thinking the word *relax*, consciously allow a certain part of your body to relax. Relax one part during each breathing cycle. Go from your head to your arms, hands, chest, abdomen, back, waist, buttocks, legs and finally your feet, in that order. After the muscles of your entire

body have been relaxed, mentally suggest to your blood vessels, nerves and internal organs that they also relax.

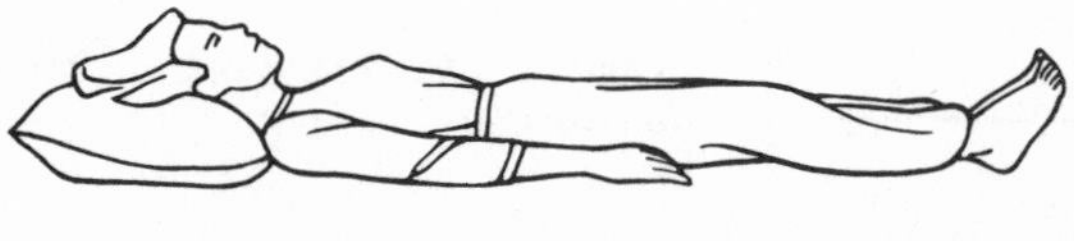

To help you remember the technique, Chinese doctors offer the following relaxation poem.

The Poem of *Fang Sung Kung*

With a high pillow I lie on my bed;
I keep my body comfortable and relaxed.
I breathe in and out naturally,
And say the word *quiet* and *relax* silently.
I think of the word *quiet* as I inhale,
And the word *relax* as I exhale.
As I silently say the word *relax*,
I tell my muscles to relax.
First, I relax my head, arms and neck,
Then my chest, abdomen, waist and back.
Finally, I tell my legs and feet to become
    relaxed.
After repeating this three times to get my body
    at ease,
I tell all my organs and cavities to relax.
I keep my breathing rhythm steady, narrow
    and even
While focusing my attention on my abdomen.
As my mind enters into a state of mental
    quietness,
I enjoy this sleeplike but awake state of
    consciousness.
After I stay in this state for a short period
    of time,
I rub my face, get up, move around and
    feel fine.

Figure 38. *Supine position for relaxation breathing exercises*

Ch'iang Chuang Kung — Invigorating Breathing

Ch'iang Chuang Kung, the invigorating breathing exercise, can be used to treat diseases such as anxiety and depression, high blood pressure, heart disease and emphysema. *Ch'iang Chuang Kung* pays special attention to *ju ching*, the method of entering into the state of mental quietness. It is not as demanding as some other types of *Ch'i Kung* in requirements for regulating the breathing rhythm.

In this form, an ordinary sitting position is most often used. You can also adopt the cross-legged or standing position. The physically weak may use a lying-down position.

The recommended position is sitting straight on a balanced stool or chair of comfortable size. Place both feet firmly on the ground, a shoulder width apart. Your knees should form a 90-degree angle and your body should be straight. Your thighs and trunk should also form a 90-degree angle.

Place your hands, palms down, gently on your legs. Allow your elbows to bend naturally. Keep your head, waist and back straight. Allow your shoulders to fall naturally. Let your chest and chin turn slightly inward. (See Fig. 39.) The requirements for your eyes, mouth and tongue are the same as those in *Fang Sung Kung*. (See page 44.)

Alternatively, you can adopt a natural cross-legged position. Sit steadily on a cushion with your legs crossed, your feet under your legs, your knees off the floor and your buttocks sticking slightly out behind you. Keep your waist and back straight and your chest curved slightly in. Allow your shoulders to drop naturally. Keep your head straight but turn your chin slightly inward.

Place one hand on top of the other near your navel or on your abdomen with your thumbs crossing each other. (See Fig. 40.) Your eyes, mouth and tongue follow the same standards as for *Fang Sung Kung*. (See page 44.)

Of standing positions, the so-called three round style is the most desirable. However, this

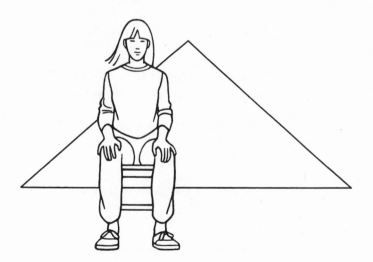

Figure 39. *Mental quietness before invigorating breathing*

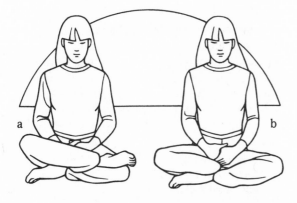

Figure 40. *Cross-legged breathing poses*

minute. Although the duration of each breathing cycle is lengthened, your breathing must still be natural and relaxed. Never tense your muscles or apply force. Never attempt to breathe deeply through unnatural effort.

Ju ching, entering mental quietness, is the key here. The fundamental principle of *Ch'iang Chuang Kung* is to focus *yi*, your consciousness, on your lower abdomen.

In the beginning, you may develop the habit of concentration by silently counting or mentally following the movement of each breathing cycle. Through practice, you will eventually learn to passively focus attention on your lower abdomen without effort.

To use the breath counting method, silently count each time you inhale and exhale. Count

position is appropriate only for relatively healthy persons. To assume it, stand with your feet a shoulder width apart, your toes pointing slightly inward and your knees slightly bent. Keep your waist straight, your chest flat and your arms raised. Hold your arms in front of you, approximately at shoulder level, as if you were embracing a large tree. Your elbows may be somewhat lower than your shoulders. Bend your fingers as if your hands held an imaginary ball. (See Fig. 41a.)

In this position, you can use either natural breathing or abdominal deep breathing. Breathing naturally, you just breathe in and out through your nose as in *Fang Sung Kung*.

With abdominal deep breathing, your abdomen will swell naturally as you inhale and contract as you exhale. If you want, place your hands on your abdomen as in Fig. 41b. You should gradually increase the depth of each inhalation and exhalation until the number of your breathing cycles is reduced to 6 to 8 per

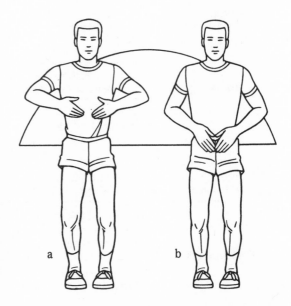

Figure 41. *Standing breathing poses*

from one to ten and then back to one again. If you lose track of the counting because of mental distractions, just start the counting over again.

Focusing on your breathing is a more natural method than counting breaths. Just allow your thoughts gently to follow the movement of each breathing rhythm. Keep your attention on your breathing. If distractions occur, recall your thoughts and place them on the movement of each breath.

The *yi* focusing method, another way of getting mentally quiet, involves thinking of the energy center *Tan Tien*, which is approximately 3 inches below your navel. The idea is to place your thoughts very gently and easily on this spot without trying. Do not force yourself to concentrate. Let it be completely natural. If distractions do occur, return your thoughts to the same spot again. You should practice *Ch'iang Chuang Kung* as often and for as long as you would *Fang Sung Kung*.

The following table summarizes an orderly progression for developing your practice of *Ch'iang Chuang Kung*.

Table 1

A Chart for the Practice of *Ch'iang Chung Kung*

Step #	1 *(1st week)*	2 *(2d to 4th weeks)*	3 *(5th week and thereafter)*
Posture	Lying or regular sitting position	Regular sitting or cross-legged sitting position	Sitting or standing position
Breathing	Natural breathing progressing to moderate deep breathing	Natural deep breathing (abdominal type)	Natural deep breathing (abdominal type)
Consciousness	Counting breaths; following breaths	Following breaths, placing *yi* on lower abdomen	Placing *yi* on lower abdomen
Frequency and Duration	3 to 4 times daily 15 to 20 minutes a time	3 to 4 times daily 30 minutes a time	3 to 4 times daily 30 to 40 minutes a time
Requirements	1. Correct posture 2. Breathing is narrow, even, steady but with latent energy 3. Eliminate mental distractions	1. Longer and deeper breathing, *ch'i* sinking into *Tan Tien* 2. Initial mental quietness 3. Practice regularly	1. Breathing is now narrow, long, deep, slow, steady, soft and even 2. Complete mental quietness 3. Improvement in health 4. Interest in *Ch'i Kung*

Nei Yang Kung—Internally Nourishing Breathing

Nei Yang Kung, the internally nourishing breathing exercise, is especially appropriate for treating gastric and duodenal ulcers, hepatitis, a general rundown condition and habitual constipation. It pays special attention to the technique of breathing itself.

For *Nei Yang Kung*, the lying-on-the-side and regular sitting positions are preferred. The supine position may also be used.

You should do the lying-on-the-side position on your right with your head bent slightly to the front. Bend your right arm beside your chest and place your hand on the pillow about 2 inches away from your head with your palm up. Stretch your left arm out naturally and place your hand on your hip, palm down. Bend both legs naturally with your left leg on top of your right leg. (See Fig. 42.) Or you may use any position that is natural and relaxing.

If you want to use the lying-on-the-back position, you'll find directions in the section on *Fang Sung Kung*, page 44.

Directions for the regular sitting position can be found in the *Ch'iang Chuang Kung* section, page 46.

Using the correct breathing method is especially important with this *Ch'i Kung*, and the method involves some new techniques. Begin by breathing in and out through your nose, using the abdominal method. Then pause for a moment between each breathing cycle. More specifically, inhale and exhale, pause and raise your tongue to the roof of your mouth and do a short silent recitation before lowering your tongue and inhaling. (Suggestions concerning your choice of a recitation follow.)

During the moment that you pause, do not tense your muscles and hold your breath. Nor should you stop the breath in your upper abdomen or throat.

In a breathing pause, what is intended is that you center your consciousness on the lower abdomen with a temporary cessation in breathing. The duration of the pause may be gradually increased as you recite more words. It takes about 1 second to recite 1 word. Most people recite between 3 and 7 words, which of course will take 3 to 7 seconds.

The phrase or sentence you choose to silently recite should have an appropriate message. For example, you could recite phrases such as "be peaceful," "good to be peaceful," or "relaxation is good for health."

The physiological effects of breathing pause need further study. But it appears that this type of breathing tends to create pressure in the abdominal cavity, which results in improved blood circulation and intestinal movement.

Ju ching, the state of mental quietness, is gradually entered when concentration is guided by coordinating your breathing with the silent recitation of a phrase or sentence. When the mind is in a state of relaxation, distractions are

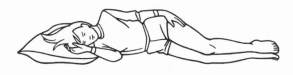

Figure 42. *A position for internally nourishing breathing*

less likely to occur. This technique is relaxing and centering. As a result, you will enter the state of mental quietness.

The Up and Down Gymnastic Breathing Exercise

The up and down breathing exercise is easy to do yet therapeutically effective. It not only helps prevent high blood pressure and bronchitis, but also helps develop fitness.

1. To prepare for this exercise, relax your entire body. Stand naturally with your feet a shoulder width apart and your arms hanging naturally. (See Fig. 43a.) Mentally concentrate on the movements as you do them slowly and evenly. Breathe naturally.

2. With your arms slightly bent, lift your hands with your fingers naturally curled over your head from the front. At the same time, breathe in. Begin inhaling as you start to lift your hands and finish inhaling when your hands are over your head. (See Fig. 43b.)

3. Next bend both knees to squat down.

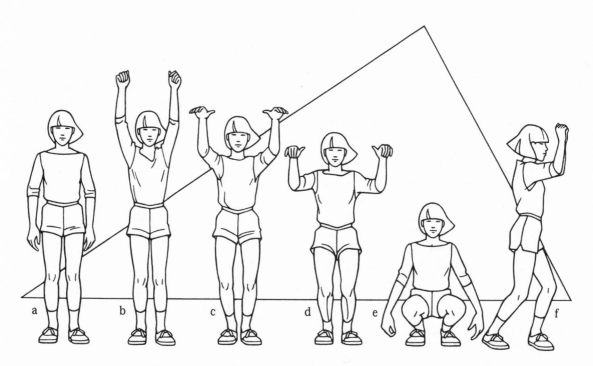

a   b   c   d   e   f

Figure 43. *The up and down gymnastic breathing exercise*

(See Fig. 43c.) Keep your upper body straight, open your hands and lower your arms to the front as you squat down naturally and exhale. (See Fig. 43d.) After your hands have been lowered, place them beside your legs. (See Fig. 43e.) Note that squatting, arm lowering and exhaling all start and finish at the same time.

4. Then rise up on your legs again as you simultaneously lift your arms to the front and over your head. As you do this, breathe in. Count each up and down movement cycle as one exercise. You may repeat it 10 to 20 times, depending on your condition. Avoid excessive repetitions as they may cause dizziness. If the number of repetitions is about right, you should feel refreshed after the exercise.

5. After you have become proficient at doing this movement, you may also rotate your body from side to side while you are in the standing position. (See Fig. 43f.) Turn your whole body to left and right. Turn your head and neck, too. This rotation should be done when your body has risen to the standing position, your arms have been lifted upward, and exhalation has begun.

To the knowledge of Chinese doctors, many persons have cured themselves of certain nagging and stubborn diseases by persistently performing this exercise.

Involving the movement of the entire body and a coordination between motion and breathing, this exercise series must be done slowly and softly with an even and long breathing rhythm. From the physiological viewpoint, it speeds up blood circulation and digestion of foods, improves ability to take in air, absorb oxygen and expel carbon dioxide, and strengthens chest and abdominal muscles, particularly the breathing muscles. Therefore, it is very suitable for chronic disease patients.

Doing *Tai Chi Rod*

Tai Chi Rod, one of many ancient Chinese fitness methods, is basically the same as *Tai Chi Chuan* in terms of its demand for relaxation, peacefulness and spontaneousness. It, too, integrates movement with mental quietness. For this reason, it is called *Tai Chi Rod* or *Tai Chi Ruler*.

Tai Chi Rod has the following characteristics and advantages. You need only simple equipment. To do this exercise all you need is a rod or stick of a foot's length. It does not matter whether it is thick or thin.

The simple movement of *Tai Chi Rod* makes it easy to achieve mental quietness. The nature of its movement also tends to induce internal placidness. Therefore, it is said that *Tai Chi Rod* is an exercise that unites motion and placidness.

It is simple to do. This exercise can be performed in either the sitting or standing position. The physically weak or sick may do it lying down. The only movement that's required is to circle your hands in front of your chest or to move them up and down.

Tai Chi Rod does not take up a lot of space. It can easily be performed at home. Before you do the exercise, you should make sure that the air is clean and the environment is quiet. The movements of *Tai Chi Rod* follow:

1. Relax your entire body. Close your eyes partially and breathe naturally. Focus *yi*, consciousness, on your lower abdomen. Just lie, sit or stand and relax quietly for a little while.

2. Press your palms against both ends of the rod, hold it in front of your abdomen, and move both your hands in front of your abdomen as if you were turning a wheel.

When performing the exercise while lying on your back, you should bend your elbows and

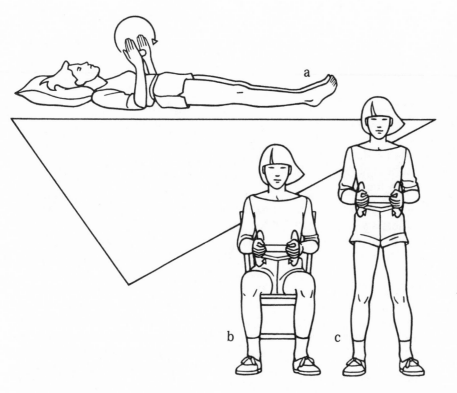

Figure 44. Tai Chi Rod
positions

keep them on the bed at all times during the exercise. Your motion, therefore, will involve pressing your palms against the ends of the rod, and swaying the rod up and down in a continuous motion. (See Fig. 44a.)

In the sitting position, you can use any posture that's comfortable. With your palms against the ends of the rod as described, bend your elbows and draw circles in front of your abdomen. (See Fig. 44b.) If you do it standing up, you should keep your feet a shoulder width apart. Draw circles in front of your abdomen as shown in Fig. 44c.

3. After you have improved your physical strength and your symptoms have lessened, you may add to these exercises, drawing circles while walking or while walking in place.

To draw circles with the rod while walking in place, you should stand with one foot in front and one foot behind. Lift one foot up and replace it on the same spot. Then do the same with the other foot. When your foot is up, draw one circle with the rod. When your foot is down, also draw one circle with the rod. Alternate which foot is in front. (See Fig. 45.)

When drawing circles while walking, you should draw one circle for each step taken. Be sure to keep your knees slightly bent at all times.

In practicing *Tai Chi Rod* you should be aware that after doing this exercise for a period of time, it is possible that you may experience a few abnormal reactions. You might feel heat and perspiration throughout your body, you may itch, your fingers might swell or your muscles may twitch. The reactions are similar to those that may be experienced when performing *Ch'i Kung*. (See page 43.)

The reactions may vary from person to person, depending on each individual's physical strength. Some people may have strong reactions. Others may have only mild reactions. Some may not have any reactions at all except for a relaxed and upbeat feeling.

You should also know that the movement of *Tai Chi Rod* will accelerate stomach and intestinal movement. While doing this exercise, you may hear noises coming from your intestines and feel the urge to break wind. You may also find your appetite significantly improved.

Practice time is usually set at 2 to 5 minutes in the beginning. After 20 to 30 days, you may increase the practice time to 5 to 10 minutes.

After another 1 to 2 months, you may increase it to 10 to 20 minutes. Do not increase the time from this point on. You may practice *Tai Chi Rod* 2 or 3 times a day.

The requirements of *Tai Chi Rod* are basically the same as those of *Tai Chi Chuan*. You may want to review the sections on *Tai Chi Chuan* or read other books on *Tai Chi Chuan*.

The movements of *Tai Chi Rod* must be soft and slow, comfortable and natural. The exercise load should be increased in a gradual manner. Do not try to accomplish everything in one day.

People of ancient times believed that practicing *Tai Chi Rod* would cure a variety of diseases. Modern experimental research suggests, however, that it is mainly helpful in the prevention of stomach and intestinal diseases such as gastric ulcers, duodenal ulcers and other digestive complaints. It's also been found helpful for anxiety, depression and high blood pressure. It is fair to say, too, that it improves overall health.

Tai Chi Rod is not appropriate, however, when you are suffering from any acute disease, fever or bleeding.

The Ancient Art of *Tsa Fu Pei*—Knocking at the Gate of Life

Tsa Fu Pei means to knock the abdomen and back. It's an ancient fitness method with the distinctive feature of combining massage, knocking and waist exercise. *Tsa Fu Pei* is effective and easy to do, and it can be performed anywhere.

According to traditional Chinese medical theory, the area located 3 inches below the navel is so important that it's called *Tan Tien* or *Ch'ien Ming Men*, the Front Gate of Life. The corre-

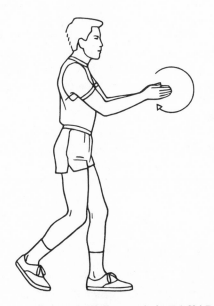

Figure 45. *Walking with the* Tai Chi Rod

sponding position on the back is *Ming Men*, Life Gate, or *Hau Ming Men*, the Back Gate of Life. Because this exercise involves knocking in the vicinity of the *Ming Men* acupuncture point, it is also called "knocking at the gate of life." Here's how to do *Tsa Fu Pei*:

1. Relax your entire body. Bend your knees slightly and make loose fists. Let your arms hang down naturally. Focus *yi*, consciousness, on your navel.

2. Start by placing your loose fists against your front and back life gates. Then turn your body at the waist to start your arms swinging. Let one loose fist strike just below your navel as the other hits the *Ming Men* region of your back. (See Fig. 46.) While turning at the waist to the

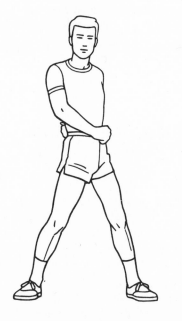

Figure 46. *Knocking at the gate of life*

left and to the right, keep in mind that your arms should swing like ropes, without the slightest effort, and your hands and fists should act like hammers. The knocking should be induced by the natural force of your turning motion, not by the stiff force of your arms.

Remember that to create the natural force of the knocking, you should loosen your entire body and rely on your waist as the axis of the rotation. Special attention should be given to relaxing your arms.

The frequency and duration of the knocking may be determined on the basis of your condition. If the exercise load is about right, you should feel relaxed and comfortable and perspire a little.

Do not do this exercise immediately after a meal. It should be done one or more hours after eating. The best time to do it is in the morning when there is plenty of fresh air.

Keep your breathing natural. You may breathe with only your nose or with both your nose and mouth at the same time.

The knocking will vibrate your internal organs. The vibrations will help improve your digestion and speed up blood circulation. Apply force in a step-by-step progressive manner, however. Do not overreach yourself by increasing the exercise load too fast.

This exercise is relatively effective in increasing physical strength. However, further study needs to be done to determine for which diseases this exercise is most appropriate.

Li Shou—What Hand Swinging Can Do for You

Li Shou, the hand swinging exercise, has been passed down from generation to generation by the common people of China. It did not originate from *Yee Chin Ching* as some have claimed.

Li Shou is well known for its effectiveness in increasing physical strength and building up resistance to disease. It is also therapeutically useful in treating certain chronic diseases such as bronchitis, stomach and intestinal diseases, high blood pressure, depression and anxiety.

However, it is certainly not a panacea for all kinds of diseases as some have been led to believe. The phrase *Li Shou* therapy should not be used because *Li Shou*, like other exercises such as *Tai Chi Chuan* and *Pa Tuan Chin*, is only one approach to physical fitness. But it is a special one.

The movement of *Li Shou* is simple and easy to do. It can be performed anytime. It is especially suitable for the elderly and physically weak as well as for patients with chronic diseases in general. You can vary the number of swings per session and the number of sessions per day to suit yourself and your condition.

As with other fitness methods, you should proceed step by step, increasing the number of swings only gradually. You should not get the idea that the more you swing the better. In fact, swinging for too long may do more harm than good.

If done properly, *Li Shou* can usually help patients with various chronic diseases improve their appetites, increase their physical strength, build up their resistance to disease, lessen symptoms, sleep better and sometimes even cure their diseases.

When practicing *Li Shou*, you must maintain a comfortable and natural posture, keep your movements loose and follow the correct method persistently. You should increase your repetitions only gradually. If you ignore your health and perform *Li Shou* with the wrong idea that the more swings the better, and the more force the better, then you may experience some side effects with possibly harmful consequences.

In the process of being handed down from generation to generation, *Li Shou* has evolved into more than ten variations. The following is one of the most fundamental and popular varieties, known to have among the best healing effects.

Begin by standing still with your feet a shoulder width apart. Keep your body straight and let your arms hang down naturally. Look straight ahead. Make sure that you feel comfortable.

Keep your neck loose and your face natural throughout the exercise. Put on a happy face—it will help you become relaxed. Close your mouth and let your lips and teeth gently touch. Let your tongue lay flat.

Keep your spine relaxed but upright, your chest straight but comfortable. Do not thrust your chest forward. Keep your waist and stomach loose. Don't stick your stomach out. When these requirements are met, you will naturally feel heavy and full in the abdomen.

Keep your shoulders loose and let them hang down. Let your arms hang, too. Don't straighten your elbows. Do not hold your arms tightly against your body. Leave some space under your armpits. Keep your fingers naturally apart—do not intentionally bend or straighten them. Keep your palms slightly bent and facing toward your sides.

Place your toes, soles and heels firmly and evenly on the ground, with your toes pointing forward. Your clothes and belt should be loose.

In the position just described, relax your body and calm your mind for 1 or 2 minutes. After your mind has calmed down, you may start swinging your hands fluidly from front to back.

When your arms are out in front your thumbs should not be higher than the navel. When your hands are being swung back, the outer edges of your little fingers should not go higher than your buttocks. When you are ready, swing your hands back and forth.

Guidelines for *Li Shou*

Your entire body must be relaxed, particularly your shoulders, arms and hands. Relaxation will facilitate the circulation of *ch'i* (energy) and blood, and cause blood and *ch'i* to flow downward. This way your lower body will become heavy and firm. While swinging your hands, you should have a feeling known in China as empty-top-but-solid-bottom.

Your hand swing should be accompanied by the movement of your waist and legs. Do not just swing your arms. Waist movement can help strengthen your internal organs and thus produce greater effects.

Your breathing should be natural. Do not make a deliberate attempt to coordinate hand movement with breathing rhythm. Greater benefits can be obtained when you learn gradually to breathe with your abdomen.

Your arms should be as loose as a rope. Your fingers should be separated naturally. Do not tense your muscles.

Patients who are seriously ill may swing their hands in the sitting position. However, they should be careful not to overdo it.

You should integrate movement and mental quietness. Because *Li Shou* consists of simple movements that are performed with relaxation and mental concentration, it provides a natural setup for inducing mental quietness. The effects of *Li Shou* are, therefore, similar to those of *Ch'i Kung*.

When external movement and internal quietness are fully coordinated, the external movement becomes spontaneous. The result is that you will feel good about your entire body.

If you find excessive saliva in your mouth, swallow it rather than spitting it out.

Count each back-and-forth swing as one movement. The number of movements to be performed differs from person to person. It must, however, be increased only gradually. Do not force yourself to break your own record. As you are swinging your hands, silently count the number of swings. If you prefer, you can also swing for a set amount of time.

Keep your eyes partially closed. Keep your mental focus on your navel. Unite your external movement with internal quietness. Feel heavy and firm in your lower body.

Whenever possible, perform *Li Shou* in clean air and in a quiet environment. Stop practicing when there are thunderstorms. Nor should you do *Li Shou* right after a heavy meal or when you are hungry.

When you are doing *Li Shou* right, you should feel very relaxed and comfortable during and after the exercise. If you experience any dizziness, chest pain, nausea or extreme fatigue, you should reduce the number of sessions or stop the exercise for the time being. These problems are most often caused by swinging too many times and swinging with too much force.

Do not swing too high to the front. The back swing should not be higher than the buttocks. If you ignore this advice, you may get side effects such as dizziness or fever.

After the exercise, you should remain standing for 1 or 2 minutes. Then do some relaxing exercises before returning to normal activities.

During the hand swinging, it is possible that you may feel cold or warm. Or you may hear noises coming from your abdomen or feel the urge to break wind. You may also experience the sensations of numbness, a swelling pain or insects crawling on your skin. Some people feel the *ch'i*, energy, circulating inside their bodies, and some may make involuntary movements. These are normal (but not universal by any means) physiological phenomena brought about by the integration of motion with mental quietness in *Li Shou*. The extent to which they occur varies from person to person. Some people may not have any of these reactions at all.

These happenings are similar to those that one may experience while practicing *Ch'i Kung*. You should not be overly concerned about them. There is no need to get excited nor to be afraid. Leave these sensations alone. Just let them be.

Do not make a conscious attempt to produce these reactions because they do not in themselves have any healing effect. Many people who have practiced *Ch'i Kung* for a long time have never experienced these phenomena. Nevertheless, they have obtained very much the same results as those who have had these reactions. Some people who made a special effort to pursue unusual reactions experienced nervous tension and other unpleasant symptoms.

Running for Health

As a disease prevention exercise, running has gained worldwide popularity because it is effective, yet easy to do. The benefits of fitness running —running performed primarily for improving health and preventing disease—include training and protecting your heart.

Your physical strength and endurance are related to the condition of your muscles. But more importantly, they are related to the amount of oxygen your body can absorb during exercise. The greater the amount of oxygen you can absorb, the greater your capacity for physical activity. The amount of oxygen that can be absorbed is a function of the efficiency of your heart or your cardiovascular system.

Studies indicate that running, if done properly, can strengthen your heart and improve its efficiency. A healthy and efficient heart will do a better job of helping your body absorb more oxygen. In a study in which ten subjects ran on a treadmill for 10 minutes every day for 3 months, their oxygen consumption per heartbeat was increased by almost 15 percent.

A study of another group of subjects also showed a significant increase in the level of oxygen absorption after they had run 30 minutes daily for 4 weeks at heart rates of around 150 beats per minute.

Before training, one group complained of breathlessness after running a distance of several hundred yards. But after they'd trained, these same people were able to run several miles without feeling tired. These are the beneficial effects of cardiovascular training.

Running protects the hearts of the middle-aged and elderly who are especially vulnerable to heart diseases caused by an inadequate blood supply to the heart muscle. When their coronary (heart) arteries are obstructed, their heart muscles may not get sufficient blood. The consequence may be angina pectoris—heart pain—even myocardial infarction—heart attack. But people who run over an extended period of time are less inclined to have obstructed arteries even as they get older. Systematic regular running can help insure that the heart muscle is working at optimal efficiency. And in this way, running can prevent coronary heart disease.

Running also improves circulation and has a revitalizing effect on the blood. Running speeds up circulation and alters the way blood is distributed in the entire body. When you run, the muscle groups in your legs alternately contract and relax. This action forcefully drives venous blood back to the heart. As a result it's less likely that blood will pool in your legs and pelvic cavity. This guards against thrombosis or clot formation in the veins. Running also accelerates the breakdown of fibrin—a protein normally found in the blood—into soluble fragments and stops formation of fibrin clots. Both of these factors contribute to preventing clot-clogged veins.

Running contributes to health by helping to control body weight. Overeating, coupled with physical inactivity, is the most frequent cause of overweight and obesity, which have been implicated in a number of diseases. The rates for diabetes, coronary heart disease and gallbladder disease are much higher in overweight and obese persons than in persons of average body weight. Therefore, it's important to control body weight, particularly for the middle-aged.

Running is an effective way to prevent obesity. Running speeds up metabolism, consumes energy, breaks down glycogen (blood sugar) and reduces fat storage. The rate of calorie burnoff during running is many times that of the resting rate. A healthy individual consumes about 100 calories when running 400 yards at full speed. Jogging 3 miles will burn 450 calories, about one-fifth of an average daily intake.

But underweight and weak persons with inadequate digestive functioning can also benefit from running. Running—mainly slow running —can improve their metabolic function, their appetites and their digestion. These changes should contribute to an appropriate increase in body weight.

More Reasons to Run

In addition, running improves lipometabolism, which is essentially the metabolism of fats, and helps prevent arteriosclerosis, hardening of the arteries. One of the most common causes of arteriosclerosis is the body's failure to metabolize lipids efficiently. When there is a heavy concentration of low-density lipoproteins (LDLs) in the bloodstream and too few high-density lipoproteins (HDLs), cholesterol has a tendency to deposit on the walls of the arteries. The arteries become narrow and hard—arteriosclerosis has developed.

Running, particularly regular and systematic long-distance running, can improve the metabolism of lipids and lower the blood level of LDLs and increase HDLs. Running also helps reduce serum cholesterol in the blood.

In one experimental group, tests showed that serum cholesterol fell significantly after only one session of long-distance running. Some members of the group ran about 2 miles, and some about 3, at a speed of about 8 minutes a mile.

A group of patients with high blood pressure also reduced their level of serum cholesterol by more than one-fourth after participating in a 2-year program of long-distance running.

Running has also been found to reduce the level of triglycerides, another type of fat implicated in the formation of artery-clogging plaque. One study showed that long-term consistent runners had only half the triglycerides of non-runners, as well as a lower LDL level.

It appears that running can not only prevent hyperlipemia, excess fatty substances in the blood, but as a result, can also help prevent arteriosclerosis and coronary heart disease.

Running, especially slow-paced outdoor running, can help condition the neuro-vascular system and prevent high blood pressure. Running regulates cortical activity, reduces mental fatigue and reduces emotional stress and depression.

Slow running helps desensitize the nerves

that control the activity of the heart. It can contribute to the treatment of certain functional disorders of the cardiovascular and nervous systems.

Long-distance running has a number of effects which contribute to the prevention of hypertension. It helps decrease sympathetic nerve arousal, yet excites the vagus nerve. It desensitizes smooth muscles in the small arteries and reduces the possibility that they will contract spasmodically. All of this helps prevent high blood pressure and explains why long-distance runners tend to have lower blood pressure than other people.

Even people who already suffer from moderate hypertension can sometimes lower their blood pressure with slow cautious running. There's a special section dealing with this situation beginning on page 73.

How Far, How Fast and How Often to Run

In fitness running, which is aimed at treating diseases and improving health, you should carefully determine the proper workload—the distance, speed and frequency of training sessions.

Generally speaking, short-distance fast-paced running is rarely used therapeutically. Therapeutic exercise relies primarily on slow-paced running, either long or short distances, and intermittent running, which will be discussed later.

Beginners who are physically weak may start by running at a speed of approximately 30 to 40 seconds per 100 yards. The intensity level in this type of running is very low. It is almost like fast walking.

Slow long-distance running is the most frequently used type of fitness running. You can start training at a distance of about ½ mile. Once you have adapted well to this distance, you may add ½ mile to your workload each week or every other week until your total is between 1½ and 3½ miles.

Intermittent running—alternating slow-paced running with walking—is a style that suits those with weak hearts and lungs. In order to avoid overburdening the heart, you should start by running 30 seconds and follow it by walking for 60 seconds. Repeat this sequence 20 to 30 times. The whole session should last 30 to 45 minutes. The speed of your running may be varied, depending on your level of health and fitness.

With short-distance slow-paced running and with intermittent running, a once-a-day or once-every-other-day frequency is desirable. With slow long-distance running, young physically fit persons may run 30 minutes a day, 3 to 5 days a week. Older, less fit individuals should do 20 to 30 minutes of running a day, 2 or 3 times a week.

To get the best results, a runner should strive to reach the maximum permissible level of intensity. This differs from person to person and may be determined on the basis of the heart rate, age and level of fitness. Individuals who are basically physically fit may use this simple formula as a guide to calculating their maximum level of intensity: 180 minus their age. The following table shows maximum recommended heart rate (beats per minute) for different age groups.

Age	30–39	40–49	50–59	60–69
Maximum Heart Rate (beats/min.)	182	178	167	164

To get a more precise figure for optimal rate during running, subtract your resting heart rate from your maximum rate given in the table. Multiply this number by 60 percent, then add your resting heart rate.

For example, suppose we have a 48-year-old man who is healthy and has average physical strength. If his heart rate at rest is 76 beats per minute, then the formula to determine his optimal running heart rate will be: $178 - 76 \times 60\% + 76 = 137.2$, or 137.

For patients with chronic diseases and weak hearts and lungs, the following formula to determine optimal running heart rate should be used instead. Subtract the patient's age from 170. Thus, the optimal heart rate for a 48-year-old chronic disease patient with a weak heart would be figured: $170 - 48 = 122$.

It should be emphatically pointed out that the so-called optimal exercising heart rate is provided for reference only. No one should rigidly adhere to it. The intensity level of any exercise should be based on your particular condition, including your health status and your training background. If the exercise workload is about right, you should generally feel comfortable, energetic and be able to eat and sleep well.

Rules for Running

Certain rules must be followed when running is used for improving health and preventing disease. Patients with chronic diseases in particular should take certain precautions.

The first and most obvious requirement is that the patient should determine whether or not to run at all. Those who may run include healthy middle-aged or elderly persons who run to *prevent* coronary heart disease, hypertension and hyper-lipemia (high levels of blood fats) or to control their body weight and improve their health.

Patients who *have* hyperlipemia, suspected coronary heart disease, stabilized coronary heart disease or borderline hypertension may run as a form of therapy if they do so cautiously, with their doctor's permission.

Chronic disease patients in general, if they have adequate physical strength, may run to increase their strength and improve their heart and lungs.

But anyone in the acute stage of a disease should not run. Nor should most patients with cirrhosis, pulmonary tuberculosis or severely arthritic legs. Untreated metabolic diseases such as diabetes, hyperthyroidism, hypothyroidism, myxedema (another thyroid-related disease), or serious anemia where the hemoglobin count is very low or a susceptibility to bleeding are all conditions that preclude running.

Patients suffering from certain cardiovascular diseases also should not run. Those who have serious valvular disease, who had a recent heart attack, who have recurrent angina pectoris, the onset of ventricular tachycardia, untreated atrial fibrillation, cardiomyopathy, second- or third-degree heart block, myocarditis or congestive heart failure are also forbidden to run.

For the sake of safety, even healthy middle-aged people should have medical checkups before running. And chronic disease patients should not engage in running without first consulting their physician.

Patients with chronic diseases should carefully monitor their own physical reactions when practicing long-distance running. Special attention should be paid to changes in pulse rate or any increase in symptoms. A periodic medical checkup is also advisable.

If you have a common cold, fever or diarrhea, stop running until you feel better. Some women prefer not to run during menstruation.

Everyone should train gradually, beginning with slow short-distance running. If you adapt well to this type of running, you can slowly increase both distance and speed. But do not go beyond your own limit. Never overreach yourself and overburden your heart or become extremely fatigued.

When you do run, maintain a smooth breathing rhythm. It's a good idea to coordinate your running with your breathing. Breathe in once every two steps and exhale once every two steps. Or if it works out better for you, inhale and exhale on a count of three steps. You can breathe through both your nose and mouth at the same time.

The best time for running is in the morning, preferably after some warm-up exercises. If you can't find time in the morning, you may run in the afternoon. It is generally not desirable to run just before bedtime.

Sunbathing the Chinese Way

Plainly speaking, taking a sunbath is simply a matter of exposing yourself to the sun. Sunbaths usually come in two forms. There's the one that takes place naturally during your daily living, work and physical activities. The other must be contrived with a specific style and method.

There are several advantages to be gained from sunbathing. For one thing, the sun's ultraviolet radiation can stimulate the excitatory process and increase the activity of the central nervous system. This stimulates the functioning of organs throughout your body. This is why after exposure to the right amount of sunlight, most people will typically feel more energetic and cheerful.

The sun's radiation, particularly the ultraviolet portion, is powerful enough to kill bacteria and helps the body build up immunity.

Ultraviolet radiation facilitates the activation of vitamin D in the body, which assures the normal absorption of calcium and phosphorus. Sufficient calcium is essential to bone development. So, sunlight helps prevent rickets and bone disease. In proper amounts, it is especially beneficial to infants and children.

Sunlight helps condition the neural center which regulates body temperature. As a result of this conditioning, your body will be better able to adapt to high external temperatures and excessive heat.

Sunlight can also affect the activity of the heart and speed up circulation of the blood and lymph. It increases the volume of blood pumped out of one ventricle of the heart in a single beat and the total volume of air breathed per minute. It both slows and deepens the breathing rhythm.

Sunbathing can be used as one of the therapeutic means for treating the following common diseases:

Inactive pulmonary tuberculosis

Depression

Cardiovascular system diseases (when compensatory function is adequate)

Arthritis (rheumatoid arthritis at the chronic stage)

Rickets

Chronic enteritis or intestinal inflammation.

Patients should not engage in sunbathing if they have any of the following conditions:

Diseases in the acute or subacute stage

Fever

Skin inflammation

Extreme fatigue or insomnia

Susceptibility to bleeding

Certain types of pulmonary tuberculosis
that are of short duration, are in an
unstabilized condition or in which
there is inadequate compensatory
function

Serious anemia.

The Perfect Sunbath

Sunbaths come in two forms—the planned and
the unplanned. Planned sunbaths often take place
at the beach, in a swimming pool, in your back-
yard or on a balcony. Your body may be partially
or completely exposed to the sunlight. Depending on your reasons for sunbathing, you may
choose either a partial or a complete sunbath.

A partial sunbath may be employed to relieve
joint diseases, muscle pain or nerve pain. The
sunbath can help the treatment process and
lessen the pain. When taking a partial sunbath,
you should expose only the affected region to the
sunlight. Cover the other parts of your body with
a cloth, clothing or towels. This type of sunbathing
rarely triggers malignant reactions in the whole
body. It is appropriate and beneficial for the
physically weak.

For the sick and weak, the normal procedure
is to first expose a certain part of the body to
sunlight, then gradually expand the area of
exposure. The amount of time should also be
increased gradually, from 10 minutes or so to 1

to 2 hours, depending on your condition. If the
exposure period is long, you may take several
breaks in a shady area.

The unplanned sunbath takes place during
your daily living, work or physical activities and
requires no special preparation.

When taking a sunbath, you should select a
place that is dust free so that dust will not interfere
with the ultraviolet radiation. The ideal location
for sunbathing is the beach, in the mountains
or in a place near a river or lake. The sunlight
contains a greater amount of ultraviolet rays in
these areas.

You should not take a sunbath on an empty
stomach or right after a meal. Also, don't eat
until 20 or 30 minutes after your sunbath.

A planned sunbath is best taken while lying
down. Cover your head with a white towel, or a
straw or bamboo hat. Also, it is desirable to protect your eyes by wearing dark glasses.

During a sunbath, do not sleep, read or
smoke. After your sunbath, rest under a shady
tree for 10 minutes or more. Afterward, take a
shower or rub your body.

During sunbathing, if you find reddish
spots on your skin or feel a burning, itching or
painful sensation, you should immediately stop
the sunbath.

If after taking a sunbath, you develop a headache, insomnia, an increased heart rate, indigestion or experience weight loss, then you should
stop sunbathing. It may be better for you to rest
for a few days without any sunbaths. Or you may
simply want to reduce the exposure time.

The best time of day for sunbathing will
vary according to geographical regions and seasons. The ideal time is usually between 9 and 12
A.M., and 4 and 6 P.M. If the sunlight is very
strong, you may stay in a shady area to receive
indirect radiation.

The Benefits of Cold Water Bathing

Cold water bathing can condition blood vessels and nerves to better adapt to external temperature changes. This can help prevent the common cold.

Cold water first stimulates the skin. Your skin has many peripheral nerve endings and a network of blood vessels which contain one-third of the blood in the entire body. Cold water training increases your body's ability to tolerate cold by improving the capacity of the blood vessels in the skin to react and respond.

Cold water stimulation of the skin produces three levels of reaction. In the first, skin blood vessels constrict. The skin turns pale and goose bumps appear.

In the second stage following constriction, the blood vessels in the skin start to dilate and allow blood to flow to the body surface from the internal organs. The color of the skin changes from pale to light red. You feel warmth all over your body.

Cold water bathing usually produces the changes of both the first and the second stage. However, if the water temperature is too low or the stimulation lasts too long, or if your body does not respond properly to the stimulation, the nerves of the blood vessels may fail to react properly. They continue to dilate and too much blood is released in a confined area. The skin turns purplish red or purplish blue. Your entire body feels cold. This is the reaction of the third stage and should be avoided.

The physiological responses of the skin blood vessels to temperature changes are governed by the vasomotor reflex that presides over the dilation and contraction of the vessels.

Frequent cold water bathing can help the body prepare for the stimulation of low outdoor temperatures. It can also increase the responsiveness of the nerves of the blood vessels so that they can adapt rapidly to sudden changes in temperature. This will protect your body from cold-induced illnesses. This is why people who engage in cold water bathing rarely catch colds.

Cold water bathing can condition your central nervous system. It has an excitatory and invigorating effect. By increasing neural activity and exciting the central nervous system, it can reduce or remove cerebral inhibition.

In the mentally tired, the emotionally inhibited and listless depressives, a brief moment of cold water bathing can revitalize mental spirits and enhance the mood.

When your tiredness results from physical or mental overwork, a cold water bath or shower of short duration can reduce your fatigue and increase your job efficiency. Frequent cold water bathing can revitalize the whole nervous system.

Cold water bathing can also condition the digestive organs and accelerate metabolism. Because it promotes blood circulation in the abdomen, stimulates the smooth muscles of the stomach and intestines, increases stomach and intestinal movement and improves digestive functions, cold water stimulation also acts to facilitate the body's metabolic process.

Cold Water Bathing for Everyone

Cold water bathing is available in many forms. Listed in order of effectiveness from lowest to highest, they are rubbing yourself with cold water, washing with cold water, showering, taking a tub bath and winter swimming. Of these, winter swimming has the strongest effect.

Cold water bathing should start with the simplest form. First rub your body with cold water. Then wash your body with cold water. After a period of adaptation, you may switch to showering or tub bathing. Those who are physically fit may swim during the autumn and winter. Those who are physically weak may use the rubbing and washing techniques all year long.

When using rubbing and washing, the temperature of the water and the time spent doing it may be varied from person to person and from location to location. Generally speaking, the colder the water is, the shorter the bathing time should be. For example, with extremely cold water, 10 seconds to 1 minute may be enough. Before and after cold water bathing, you should engage in exercise such as running to warm up your body.

Generally speaking, patients suffering from functional nervous disorders, habitual constipation, metabolic diseases, stabilized pulmonary tuberculosis with adequate compensatory function or the merely weak in general will benefit from cold water bathing. However, patients with fever, acute or subacute diseases or serious heart disease should not take cold water baths.

Do not take a cold water bath on an empty stomach or right after a meal. And wait at least 1 hour after a meal before you take a cold outdoor swim. After your cold water bath, rest 10 or 20 minutes before eating.

Start cold water bathing during the warmer seasons. If you don't have any abnormal reactions, you can take cold water baths all year long.

If you are sweating, you should make sure that you have stopped and wiped yourself dry before engaging in cold water bathing. After strenuous exercise, you should rest for a while to allow your pulse and breathing to return to normal before taking a cold water bath.

If you feel icy cold and shivery before taking the bath, you should do some extra preparatory exercise to warm up your body. Then after you have warmed up, proceed with cold water bathing.

Keep track of your response to cold water bathing. Note your feelings, body weight, sleep habits and appetite. If you lose weight, your appetite fails or you have sleeping problems, you should stop the program for the time being.

Bathing in the Air

Air bathing refers to exposing your body to air of different temperatures. Air baths can also vary, depending on wind, humidity and the electric charge in the air.

Air baths are often classified by temperature. Cold air baths are those that vary from 49° to 57°F. Cool air baths are between 58° and 70°F. Moderate are between 71° and 77°F, warm 79° to 85°F, and hot 85°F and above.

However, to train your body, you should concentrate on cold and cool air baths. These types of air baths are similar to cold water baths in their physiological effects, except that air baths are milder.

Air baths can also excite the nerves and promote stomach and intestinal movement. After taking an air bath, you should feel more vigorous, have a better appetite, and be able to sleep well. In addition, negative ions in the air have a beneficial effect on the metabolic process as well as on the central nervous system, the respiratory system and the circulatory system.

An air bath can be planned. Wearing minimal clothes, you can receive an air bath outdoors or indoors with the windows open. It is generally a good idea for you to also do appropriate physical exercise while taking an air bath, such as walking in a circle.

You may take an air bath during the course of your daily living—while going to or returning from work or school, for instance. When receiving your air bath, try to wear thin clothes.

In the beginning, take a warm air bath. After you have adapted to that, you may gradually switch to cooler and finally to cold air baths.

The duration of the bath may also be increased gradually, depending on your condition. It is usually about right if it does not cause you to feel cold or to shiver.

The best time to plan to take a cool or cold air bath is when there is sunlight and when the air has been warmed by ultraviolet rays. Both air bath and sun bath may be taken at the same time.

When it is windy and the temperature is low, you should take your air bath during physical exercise. Most people do not take air baths when it is very windy and foggy.

In terms of health, the indications and contraindications for cool and cold air bathing are the same as those for cold water baths. These are given on page 63.

Eye Exercises Can Help Prevent Nearsightedness

The use of eye exercises and self-massage to protect the eyesight was widespread in ancient China. According to historical accounts, the most common techniques were:

1. Turning the eyeballs to the left and then to the right 7 times, closing the eyes tightly for a while, then suddenly opening them wide.

2. Pressing the center of the small excavation that lies just under the middle of the center of the eyebrow 27 times.

3. Pressing the same concavity with the joint of the thumb 36 times. Also pressing the spot between the inner corner of the eye and the nose bridge 36 times.

In recent years, a number of new eye protection exercises have been developed in China based on the idea that nearsightedness in adolescents is often a result of the improper use of the eyes. For instance, the habit of holding reading material too close to the eyes can cause eyestrain, or it can trigger spasmodic contractions in the eyelid muscles. As a result, the lens of the eye may thicken because it is temporarily pulled out of shape. This kind of nearsightedness is called pseudonearsightedness. The refraction angles have not yet been permanently lengthened.

Massaging the acupuncture points around the eyes can prevent nearsightedness because it improves the adaptability of the eye muscles, reduces spasm and improves circulation.

Can eye protection exercises help cure nearsightedness once it is established? In adult nearsightedness, exercise cannot be of much help because the refraction angles have already permanently lengthened. However, for pseudonearsightedness in children and adolescents, eye protection exercises definitely have therapeutic value. Of course, adults can also practice these exercises as a way to protect their eyes.

In order to prevent nearsightedness, children and adolescents, in addition to performing eye protection exercises, should frequently engage in a variety of physical exercises and should practice good eye habits, such as holding reading material a proper distance from their eyes.

Here are some frequently recommended eye protection exercises:

1. With your eyes closed, gently rub with your thumbs the *T'ien Yin* acupuncture point,

which lies between the eyebrow and the upper corner of the orbital cavity—the bony structure that surrounds the eye. (See Fig. 47.)

2. Squeeze and press the *Ching Ming* points which lie just beyond the inner corner of the eye on the nose. Use your thumb and index finger. First press downward, then squeeze upward.

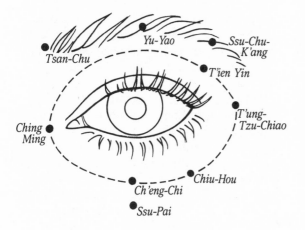

Figure 47. *Eye acupuncture points*

3. Knead your *Ssu-Pai* point. Here's how to find it. First, press your index and the middle fingers together, then place them on the sides of the bridge of your nose. Your thumbs will naturally fit against your lower cheek bones. Without removing your thumbs from your cheeks, let your index fingers find the spot on the bone right below the lowest portion of your eye socket. Curl your other fingers out of the way and

knead gently. Use your thumbs to rub the *T'ai-Yang* point. (It's not shown in Fig. 47, but it's in that hollow right below the end of your eyebrow.) Then curl your index finger and use the side of the second joint to rub all the way around your eye socket, beginning at the top near your nose. By doing this, you massage several acupuncture points, such as *Tsan-Chu, Yu-Yao, Ssu-Chu-K'ang, T'ung-Tzu-Chiao* and *Ch'eng-Ch'i* at the same time.

Eye protection exercises can be done 1 or 2 times a day. Repeat each massage 20 to 30 times. Try to rub the acupuncture points as accurately as possible. The movement should be gentle and slow. Stop massaging when there is a sensation of numbness in the area.

Hair Loss and Therapeutic Exercise

The reasons for baldness are quite complicated. It may be related to heredity, anemia, iron deficiency, drugs, chemotherapy, autoimmune disease or reaction, or general deterioration of health. No satisfactory treatment has yet been found for hair loss.

While potentially useful techniques to prevent baldness are being investigated, certain Chinese practices have been found to be helpful in preventing hair loss caused by health-related problems.

You can massage your scalp. Some ancient Chinese medical practitioners suggested scalp massage could prevent baldness and retard the graying of hair. Modern medicine says that massaging the scalp can indeed stimulate hair follicles and promote normal hair growth. Massage can also remove sebum or dandruff-forming oil and sloughed-off skin cells and their unhealthy effects. The following massage techniques can be used:

1. The pointing and rapping method employs your fingertips to tap and rap every spot on your head 50 to 100 times.

2. Next, rub and knead your scalp with your fingertips 50 to 100 times.

3. For hair pulling, hold a small bunch of your hair between your thumb and index finger in each hand and gently pull it downward swiftly but carefully. Do this 20 to 30 times with each clump.

For hair loss, you can also practice *Nei Yang Kung* or *Ch'iang Chuang Kung*, the internally nourishing and the invigorating deep breathing methods. (See page 46.) Generally improved health through *Ch'i Kung* can often lead to more healthy hair growth.

In the distant past a sage introduced an "upward focusing" method for preventing gray hair. This is how you do it. While practicing *Ch'i Kung*, mentally focus on nothing but the *Pai-Hui* acupuncture point, which is located in the exact middle of the flat part of your head. Whether or not this method is useful awaits further investigation.

Some people, as a result of applying massage and *Ch'i Kung*, have undoubtedly reversed the trend toward hair loss. In some individuals, new hair was found on the previously bald spot. You can expect better results if you pay attention to your diet as well as using the techniques just described. People who have anemia and iron deficiency should try vitamin B_{12}, folic acid and iron supplements. They should also be evaluated by a physician. Those who have an excessive greasy secretion (sebum) on their scalp should try vitamin B_6 and cystine, Chinese doctors recommend.

EDITOR'S NOTE: Never use large amounts of any nutrient without the supervision of your doctor.

CHAPTER THREE

Combating Heart and Circulatory Disease

康

More than a century ago in Germany, the sight of a young overweight physician repeatedly walking up and down a low hill inspired the curiosity of an onlooker. Why was he behaving in such a strange way, the doctor was asked.

The physician replied that he was taking care of his body. He told the onlooker that the hill-climbing was a program he had set for himself to counteract his physical deterioration. He'd become so fat, he said, that he had damaged his heart. He had been so short of breath and his legs were so swollen that he'd had to stop practicing medicine.

To deal with his symptoms, he'd come up with a program of walking up and down the hill again and again. In order not to overtax his heart and do it further damage, the program was very carefully and slowly paced with only gradual increases in effort. It was strictly structured in terms of distance traveled, speed of walking, number and incline of hills, and it had many mandatory rest periods.

The doctor told his questioner that he had already lost almost 11 pounds. And in 6 weeks, he had increased the number of steps he could take up the little hill each time from 100 to 527. Moreover, his pulse rate had returned to normal. From this experience, the doctor developed a form of therapy that can strengthen weak hearts and combat obesity. He called it pace-determined walking. It's one of the exercises we'll look at that offer possible benefits to people who have heart problems.

Who Should—and Shouldn't—Exercise

Before we make any suggestions about exercise for heart patients, we must issue an extreme caution. Whether or not a heart patient should do healing exercises is a decision that must be made with great care and with the approval of a physician. Improper exercise may do more harm than good, and the possibility that exercise may strain rather than strengthen the heart must be of concern. Nevertheless, some heart patients unquestionably can better their health and their hearts with healing exercise. If the decision is made to proceed, the patient should seek continued guidance and supervision of the exercise program from his or her doctor.

If you have any history of coronary artery disease; if you are at risk for coronary artery disease because of a history of smoking, elevated cholesterol, or a family history of heart disease; or if you are an over-35 male or over-40 female who has had a sedentary lifestyle, you should consult a physician before embarking on an exercise program.

Here's a general guide to the types of exercises suitable for patients who have various kinds of heart disease. Later, we'll get into specific exercises and an outline for a program of pace-determined walking.

Valvular disease: Frequently characterized by narrowing and incomplete closing of the mitral or aortic valves, this condition may rule out team sports, but not therapeutic exercises. If circulation is good, pace-determined walking, *Tai Chi Chuan*, badminton, table tennis and simple physical fitness exercises may be appropriate.

Congenital heart disease: This condition, which includes valvular abnormalities and defects in the heart walls or great vessels is usually diagnosed in infancy, but may be discovered during physical exercise. Symptoms include fatigue, difficulty breathing and change in facial color. Some young people with this disease should do only slow-paced relaxation exercises such as leisurely walking and *Tai Chi Chuan*. They should not engage in team sports even when their symptoms seem mild. However, many can participate in rigorous non-competitive exercise programs. Some even run marathons. If you have this problem, talk to your doctor about what's right for you.

Functional heart disease: This category includes people who display disturbances in the nervous system rather than organic defects. They may find it difficult to perform tasks requiring physical strength. They may feel fatigued and breathless quickly, and get pain in the heart region when they exercise. The heart rate at rest may exceed 90 beats per minute and occasionally be irregular. Patients with this syndrome tend to be irritable and have problems sleeping at night. They should not participate in exercises requiring swift movements. Instead, they should do simple, slow-paced exercises such as walking, *Tai Chi Chuan* and slow jogging.

Arrhythmia: This is a disturbance in the rhythm of the heart. The most common is extra systole, a premature contraction that doesn't disturb the basic beat. If it's caused by organic disease, the patient may have to avoid regular exercise. But an otherwise healthy person who occasionally experiences extra systole may continue to exercise under close observation by a health professional.

Coronary heart disease: A special section later in this chapter will be devoted to diseases that affect the arteries surrounding the heart.

Obviously people who suffer from the most serious heart diseases, such as myocardial infarction (heart attack) in the acute stage, recurring angina pectoris (acute pain in the heart region), worsening valvular disease or cardiomyopathy (serious degeneration of the heart muscle), shouldn't do exercises. If in doubt, be sure to check with your doctor.

Precautions for Exercising Heart Patients

Heart patients, first and foremost, should take great care not to overburden the hearts they are working to heal. Through being careful, the maximum benefits can be obtained from an exercise program. The amount and type of exercise should be chosen based on the condition of the heart.

Exercises intended for chronic heart patients can be divided into four categories, depending on the severity of the disease.

A. This group of patients is physically weak compared to healthy persons, but people in this group can perform their daily chores. However, they can't climb stairs or run as well as the healthy.

B. These patients can walk slowly on level ground for about 30 minutes without experiencing shortness of breath. But they can't walk fast or climb more than a few stairs.

C. This group is able to walk slowly for a few hundred steps. But the household routine is a strain. Even breathing may be difficult at times.

D. The last group comprises those in a critical stage of heart failure, where cardiac function is so impaired that fluid is building up in the lungs, and breathing is difficult.

Patients in the first two categories can enhance their blood circulation and increase their hearts' resiliency with well-planned exercises. The heart's ability to perform its task can be improved, and the more it improves the more it can benefit from a careful exercise program. The basic form of healing exercise should be pace-determined walking.

Unfortunately, patients in groups C and D can achieve only minor therapeutic effects from exercise. They should choose routines to protect the heart rather than to strengthen it. The most appropriate exercises for them are *Ch'i Kung*, simplified *Tai Chi Chuan* and walking for pleasure. Exercises are appropriate if they do not excessively speed up the pulse or in any way strain the heart.

While exercising and after, heart patients should carefully monitor their physical reactions. It is normal for the pulse rate to increase by 20 or 30 beats per minute immediately after exercise, so that needn't cause concern. However, shortness of breath, wheezing, heart palpitations, heart pain or irregular heart rhythm are signals to stop exercising immediately.

Patients who have fever should not exercise. And you should never start a workout if your resting heart rate exceeds 90 beats per minute.

School students who suffer from chronic heart ailments should also be encouraged to practice appropriate exercises to improve their condition, but these activities should be closely monitored by a health professional.

The Pace-Determined Walking Program

Pace-determined walking exercise may take place in a therapeutic clinic or on a hospital lawn. Patients recuperating at home can walk on the street, in a park, on a nearby hillside—anywhere there's little traffic and a peaceful atmosphere.

To begin, you should walk on level ground and cover a distance of no more than 300 yards. Gradually, you'll increase this distance to 500 yards (just over a quarter mile), then 1,000, 1,500 and 2,000 yards or more, depending on your condition.

Walk slowly initially—60 to 80 steps per minute—and take several breaks. As you progress, increase the speed to 80 to 100 steps per minute. Patients who are more fit may walk on a 3-degree to 5-degree upgrade for a short distance. If weather and health permit, pace-determined walking may be done every other day or even daily.

Several walking courses specifically designed for heart patients follow. These courses should be followed one at a time starting with the first. Generally speaking, you should stay on each program for a month and be able to perform it easily before moving to a higher level. Of course, it is not necessary to adhere rigidly to the distance

and speed if it is ever uncomfortable. But heart patients generally adjust well to this type of walking exercise if they follow it systematically.

First month: Walk on level ground for 200 to 600 yards at a speed of 2 or 3 minutes per 100 yards. Take a 5-minute break after completing each 100 yards.

Second month: Walk on level ground for 400 to 800 yards at a speed of 3 or 4 minutes per 200 yards. Take a 3-minute or 5-minute break after completing each 200 yards.

Third month: Walk on level ground for 800 to 1,500 yards. Complete the entire distance in 15 to 18 minutes. Take a 5-minute break midway and again at the completion of the distance.

Fourth month: Walk on level ground for 2,000 yards evenly divided into 2 sections. Complete each 1,000-yard section in 18 minutes. Follow each with a break of 3 to 5 minutes.

Fifth month: Walk on level ground for 2,000 yards. Include 2 100-yard sections with a 3-degree to 5-degree slope. Complete 1,000 yards, including the upgrade, in 20 to 25 minutes and then rest for 8 minutes. Return to the starting place in the same time, then rest again.

Practiced carefully and consistently, pace-determined walking will help those recovering from infectious diseases and from chronic heart diseases and obesity-related heart disease.

Breathing Exercises and the Heart Patient

China in recent years has treated heart disease with *Ch'i Kung*—the classic breathing exercises —with highly successful results. Congenital heart disease, high blood pressure, arteriosclerosis and arrhythmia have all been helped by *Ch'i Kung*. Of course, when these diseases are in the critical stage, breathing exercises shouldn't be tried.

Fang Sung Kung—relaxation breathing exercise—which helps muscles untense and promotes mental tranquility is best for heart patients. (See page 44 for full instructions.) It may be performed either lying down or sitting in a chair, depending on your physical condition.

The breathing rhythm should be as natural and spontaneous as possible. With each in and out breathing cycle, your body relaxes a bit more. And it builds on itself. The relaxation of your body makes your breathing more relaxed. That, in turn, further relaxes your body. With practice, you will be able to achieve a state of deep relaxation and peace. If you perform this exercise 2 or 3 times daily for about 30 minutes each session and practice faithfully, you should get good results.

The therapeutic effects of *Ch'i Kung* on the heart include relief from heart palpitations, improved breathing, diminuation of dizziness and an increase in energy. You'll be able to relax and sleep better. Your appetite will improve, and you won't tire as easily. Patients in China have achieved a healthful slowing and stabilization of their heart rates. To get these results, be sure to breathe naturally, freely and without tension when practicing *Ch'i Kung*. Tense unnatural breathing can increase the heart rate and cause dizziness. A special section on this technique begins on page 40.

How Healing Exercise Helps High Blood Pressure

Statistics show that physically active people rarely have hypertension, or high blood pressure. Data gathered in China show that athletes have only one-third the high blood pressure suffered by their less active peers. Those who perform physical labor also have a reduced incidence of high blood pressure, other figures show. And when those whose occupations are physically active do get hypertension, it usually occurs 10 to 15 years later than in those whose jobs require little activity.

One recent report published in China showed that of a group of men aged 50 to 60 who suffered high blood pressure, only 14 percent had jobs that were physically demanding. And 38 percent rarely took part in any physical activity.

But apparently exercise need not be vigorous to help prevent hypertension. A Peking study showed a connection between the practice of the gentle flowing art of *Tai Chi Chuan* and lower blood pressure. Comparing two groups of 50-year-olds to 89-year-olds, researchers found that the group who did *Tai Chi Chuan* had substantially lower blood pressure.

But in addition to preventing it, healing exercise can be used to treat high blood pressure when it's already established. Research in the last 30 years has confirmed this fact. Data collected in preparing this book has shown a majority of patients experienced relief not only from high blood pressure, but also from the related symptoms of dizziness, headache, insomnia and heart palpitations after only 1 month or so of healing exercise. Their pulse rate also tended to stabilize, and they felt more peaceful. In addition, many of their psychosomatic symptoms disappeared, and their strength improved.

Therapeutic exercise instilled confidence in these patients that they could fight against their disease. They were no longer afraid of suffering strokes or other illness. And half of these patients did not use medicine at all after they began practicing healing exercise. The rest of the patients on drug therapy prior to starting exercise obtained much better results from the combination of medicine and exercise than they had from medicine alone.

Healing exercise fights high blood pressure in a number of ways. The relaxation it produces helps counter overactivity in the cerebral cortex and vasomotor center that regulates the size of blood vessels and may cause blood pressure to rise. Physical exercise also lowers sympathetic nerve excitability, which is related to hypertension. And mild exercise, if practiced systematically, can excite the vagus nerve, which slows down the heart. Stimulation of the vagus nerve depresses arterial contractibility and causes dilation of the capillary blood vessels, lowering blood pressure, Chinese doctors believe.

Therapeutic exercise facilitates blood circulation and improves the body's adaptability. What usually happens is that during exercise, hypertensive patients' heart rate and systolic pressure rise rapidly. But consistent practice of healing exercise can help moderate those reactions. The patients can then increase their level of physical activity.

The patients who benefit the most from healing exercise, evidence suggests, are those with mild essential hypertension. Patients whose high blood pressure is caused by organic defects such as kidney disease obtain less satisfactory results.

The blood pressure of mild hypertensive patients generally fluctuates from normal to high. These patients may display symptoms of headache, dizziness, ringing in the ears and irritability. However, except for occasional palpitations and shortness of breath, they may not experience any pain around their heart. The most appropriate exercises for them are *Tai Chi Chuan, Ch'i Kung*, walking and self-massage.

After treatment with medication, the blood pressure of hypertensive patients with more severe cases usually stabilizes. But these patients may still experience headache, dizziness, ringing in the ears and insomnia, even more often and painfully. Sometimes when sitting still, they may have the sensation of spinning around in space. Chest pain due to insufficient oxygen reaching the heart muscle may be a problem. Patients at this stage should be restricted to light exercise.

Cautions for the Exercising Hypertensive

First of all, hypertensive patients who have medical complications such as serious arrhythmia, tachycardia, vasospasm or angina pectoris should not engage in therapeutic exercise unless they are supervised by a doctor.

Remember that the goal of healing exercise for you, the hypertensive, is to lower blood pressure, not to strengthen the heart. Exercises that are mild and slow are most beneficial in reaching that goal. High-intensity exercises, on the other hand, may bring about drastic changes in the heart rate and blood pressure. Headache and dizziness may also result. For this reason, hypertensive patients should not participate in exercises that raise the heart rate above 125 beats per minute.

If you have high blood pressure, you should work out a schedule that emphasizes a proper balance between activity and inactivity. People with mild hypertension should exercise about 1 hour a day, 2 or 3 times a week. In each of these sessions, 20 to 30 minutes may be devoted to more demanding exercises. People with moderate high blood pressure should limit their exercise to 30 minutes 2 or 3 days a week. Dividing the time into morning and afternoon sessions of 15 minutes each would be fine. In between workouts, stay relatively inactive.

While exercising, you should stay relaxed and avoid tensing your muscles. Breathe naturally and try not to hold your breath. Shun weight lifting and carrying heavy objects. Try to keep your head up to avoid dizziness.

Symptoms such as chest pain, headache, dizziness, arrhythmia, coughing and vomiting are signals to stop the exercise for the time being and consult your physician.

If the workout is a strenuous one, you should note your heart rate. Usually the post-exercise heart rate should return to the normal pre-exercise level 5 minutes after you've terminated the exercise.

Fatigue from exercise will almost always dissipate after 2 hours of rest. If you continue to feel tired, it may mean that the intensity level was too high and some adjustment is in order.

If you exercise indoors, make sure you do it in an open quiet space. And be sure to stay in close contact with a health professional and learn more about the principles and techniques of physical exercise.

High Blood Pressure and the Gentle Art of *Ch'i Kung*

In China no one questions the value of *Ch'i Kung*, the ancient system of breathing techniques, in lowering blood pressure. By slowing down the sympathetic nervous system, it speeds up recovery from hypertension. And *Ch'i Kung* is an ideal soother of the sympathetic nervous system. Its fundamental goals are to relax, calm and recenter energy.

There are many *Ch'i Kung* techniques. One is a simple relaxation exercise. While sitting in a chair and breathing naturally and spontaneously,

silently repeat the words *calm* and *relaxed* to yourself. Picture every part of your body relaxing, from your head to your feet. Feel the tension lessen in your nerves, heart and blood vessels.

Another easy *Ch'i Kung* technique can be done while standing with your feet a shoulder width apart, your knees slightly bent, and your back straight. Hold your arms in front of you as if you were gently holding a globe around its equator. As you breathe deeply and naturally, allow calming images to flow through your mind. You could picture a cool soothing sheet of water flowing over your body. Or imagine yourself playing in a beautiful, open outdoor space, your lungs full of good clean air and the sun on your skin. You feel serene and happy.

Physically weak patients may alternate standing and sitting breathing exercises. Gradually increase time given to the standing exercise from about 3 minutes to about 20 minutes. If you become tired, stop and take a rest. The standing exercise should not be done by patients with extremely high blood pressure.

The standing breathing exercise seems to be more effective in the treatment of high blood pressure than sitting breathing exercise. The standing position better corrects what Chinese doctors call the "loaded-on-the-top-empty-on-the-bottom" syndrome. This syndrome—characterized by a sensation of congestion and swelling in the head while the lower regions may feel sore and easily tired, and the feet may be unsteady—is common in hypertensives, according to Chinese observations.

The standing exercise helps correct this because it both stimulates the muscles of the legs and fixes the center of gravity in the lower body. The muscle contraction combined with breathing and self-suggestion, redirects the blood flow to the lower limbs, reducing congestion in the head.

Patients feel fresh and unburdened mentally. Their legs feel stronger and steadier.

The standing breathing exercise also helps recenter *ch'i*, or energy. You can mentally imagine your energy moving down from your head to your abdomen, or to the soles of your feet. Objectively, blood flow to the head decreases as the capillaries in your limbs dilate. As a result, blood pressure falls. Experimental studies have confirmed that when people concentrate on the acupuncture point 2 inches below their navel, blood flow follows and so, apparently, does energy. But on the contrary, concentration on—for instance—the tip of the nose actually raises blood pressure as well as the location of energy.

Ch'i Kung works on hypertension by inhibiting overactivity of the sympathetic nervous system while it activates the parasympathetic system. A proper balance between these parts of the autonomic nervous system helps reduce blood pressure. And through the deep tranquility experienced during practice, resistance to bothersome external distractions increases. All parts of the body become less subject to irritation.

Of course, hypertensive patients must practice *Chi Kung* systematically and regularly to get the best results. But it is not unusual for systolic blood pressure to be lowered by 16 points after just one session of exercise. The physical and mental relaxation and lowered respiratory rate —the natural result of *Ch'i Kung*—are that effective. However, it takes persistent effort to significantly improve a disturbed nervous system and achieve long-term results.

Other Exercises to Lower Blood Pressure

Tai Chi Chuan, therapeutic gymnastics, leisure walking and swimming all can help people who have hypertension. Patients who have mild cases may also jog and hike if they do so carefully.

Tai Chi Chuan: Tai Chi Chuan is an ideal exercise for hypertensive patients because of the softness of its movements and its quality of gentleness. It is totally without force or pressure. Muscle relaxation created by *Tai Chi* helps establish a conditioned relaxation reflex in the blood vessels which lowers blood pressure. After completing a set of simplified *Tai Chi Chuan*, systolic pressure usually falls 10 to 15 points.

Tai Chi Chuan generates mental concentration and produces peacefulness. Its smooth and harmonious movements are especially beneficial for hypertensive patients. Patients who are physically fit may perform the whole set of simplified *Tai Chi Chuan*. Weaker patients should do only half of it. Patients who are very weak or who have poor memories may simply practice any of the movements without necessarily following the entire sequence.

A good workout routine for hypertensive patients might include breathing exercises, relaxation techniques, gentle stretching and reaching exercises for the limbs and torso, walking and games. A few movements from *Tai Chi Chuan* could be interposed between exercises. The entire session should last 20 to 30 minutes and should be done 1 or 2 times a day in a group or individually.

Walking: Walking regularly can lower systolic blood pressure. We suggest walking on a flat surface 1 or 2 times a day at a moderate speed for 15 minutes to 1 hour, depending on your condition. Morning and early evening are both suitable times for walking.

Swimming: Swimming is a good exercise, especially during warm weather. Swim so that your body movements are slow and gentle. Animal studies show that swimming can help decrease the reactivity of the smooth muscles, lowering hypertension.

Games: Choose sports that are relaxing and do not involve extreme emotional reactions. Shooting baskets or badminton would be good.

Jogging and fast walking: The intensity level of these exercises is relatively high. A hypertensive patient's pulse rate may climb fairly high during jogging. Therefore, use caution in deciding if such an exercise is suitable for you. To be on the safe side, it may be best to start by walking for ½ or 1 mile at a speed of 16 to 20 minutes per mile. If there are no bad effects, you may switch to jogging. More about jogging can be found in Chapter Two.

Hiking: If high blood pressure is not complicated by other problems, young hypertensive patients whose disease is mild may climb hills. They might start by attempting an incline of 30 or 45 degrees for a distance of no more than 50 yards. They should follow this exertion with a rest period if fatigue results.

Exercise Prevents and Treats Hardening of the Arteries

Proper exercise can both help prevent and treat arteriosclerosis. According to several studies, physically active people are less likely to have hardening of the arteries and are less likely to develop coronary disease than people who don't exercise.

The coronary artery is, of course, one of the most important blood vessels because it supplies blood to the heart. Hardening of this artery is serious indeed. Fully 70 percent of the people who developed this disease were physically inactive, one study found.

Exercise can also prevent hardening of the arteries from becoming worse, doctors say. Exercise helps prevent and heal arteriosclerosis in at least two ways. The relief it provides from mental tension can minimize the risk of vasospasm, a condition in which vessels cramp and shut, preventing blood flow. And exercise is closely related to the level of cholesterol in the blood—it's a significant factor in lowering the level of artery-clogging cholesterol.

In a study of 57 middle-aged and older persons who had high cholesterol levels, half of them were able to lower their cholesterol levels over an 8-month program of exercise. Another group of physically inactive persons lowered their level of cholesterol in the blood after 1 to 2 hours of exercise a day for a minimum of 2 months.

The healing exercises recommended for patients with arteriosclerosis are basically the same as those for hypertensive patients, many of whom actually also have arteriosclerosis. If, however, their arteriosclerosis is severe, exercise should be lighter and the method and style simpler than those for hypertensives. Good exercises are walking for pleasure, simplified *Tai Chi Chuan*, therapeutic gymnastics and massage. The total time devoted to exercise should not exceed 45 minutes.

Walking: The best time for walking in the summer is in the morning or evening, avoiding the midday heat. Walk in a peaceful environment for 300 to 1,000 yards—about ¼ to ½ mile. This kind of slow walking will help you sleep well and improve your digestion.

Tai Chi Chuan: Depending on your physical condition, you can practice the entire set, do a half set, or just do some individual movements.

Knocking at the Gate of Life

Therapeutic gymnastics and massage: The goal in therapeutic gymnastics and massage is to improve physical condition as a whole, especially blood circulation in the limbs. The following exercises and massaging techniques have been drawn from an ancient Chinese fitness program designed primarily for the elderly. They are excellent for arteriosclerotic patients.

1. While sitting down, clench your hands into fists as you breathe in. Release the clench as you breathe out. (See Fig. 48.) Repeat 20 times.

2. Remain seated and put both hands behind your neck. Slowly and gently turn your upper body from side to side about 20 times — fewer if you feel dizzy. (See Fig. 49.)

3. Again while sitting, stretch your legs in front of you, hold on to the edge of your chair,

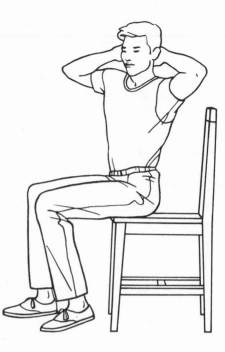

Figure 49. *Upper body turns*

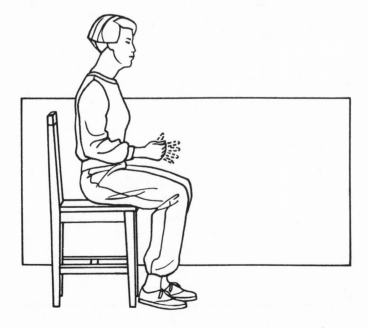

Figure 48. *Fist clenching*

and make tiny circles with your feet. (See Fig. 50.) Be sure not to overtire yourself.

4. While sitting in a chair with your back straight and your hands grasping the front edge of the seat, extend each leg, in turn, straight out in front of you. Hold it there for a few seconds. (See Fig. 51.)

5. Still sitting, stretch both legs in front of you as shown in Fig. 52, and put your hands on your thighs. Then bend at the waist and slide your hands down your legs as you breathe out. Inhale as you straighten back up. Repeat several times.

6. Massage should be done early in the morning or before bedtime; it can also be done right after exercise. Massage your head region first, rubbing your fingertips into your scalp. Then beat your shoulders with loose fists for a

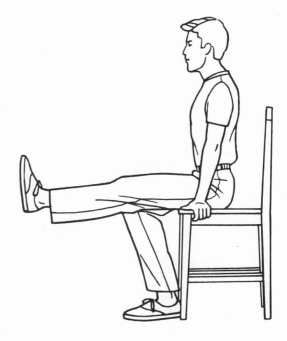

Figure 51. *Leg extensions*

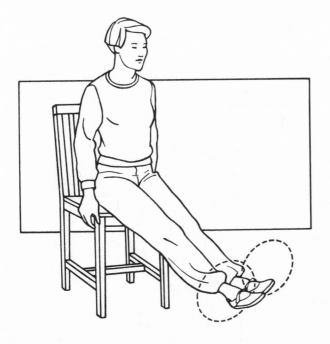

Figure 50. *Foot circling*

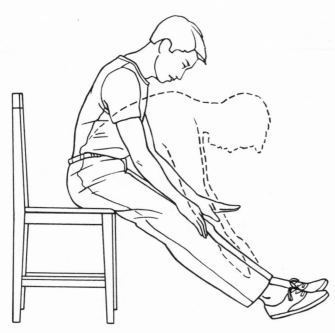

Figure 52. *Bending forward with hands on legs*

few moments, then clap your palms moderately hard on your thighs for several minutes. Fig. 53 shows a self-massage going down the arms from the shoulders—an excellent technique. Another excellent routine is clapping the legs from top to bottom—including the feet—with your open palms as you bend at the waist.

Coronary Artery Disease and Healing Exercise

Coronary artery disease, an all-too-common affliction, is characterized by a thickening of the walls of the vessels that supply the heart, reducing the flow of blood. Because of inadequate blood supply, the heart muscle doesn't get enough oxygen. The patient may feel a squeezing or pressing pain in the center of the chest, which may radiate to the arm, neck or jaw and be accompanied by shortness of breath. If the obstruction takes place suddenly, and there is a

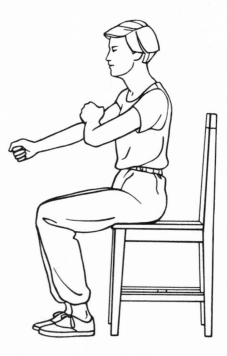
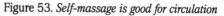

Figure 53. *Self-massage is good for circulation*

prolonged shortage of blood to the heart muscle, myocardial infarction—heart attack—results.

Physical inactivity and the onset of coronary artery disease appear to be related. Reports from China on people over age 40 show that those who frequently exercise are much less likely to have coronary artery disease than the inactive. Similar findings have been reported in other countries. Physically active persons, even when they did have heart attacks, died less frequently in the first 48 hours following the attack than their chair-bound counterparts.

There can be no doubt that frequent physical exercise helps prevent the development of coronary heart disease. In recent years, therapeutic exercises for coronary disease have been developed and used in many parts of the world with beneficial results. For patients who have not yet actually suffered heart attacks, exercise therapy can help improve fitness and speed up recovery from clogged arteries.

Physical exercise helps heal coronary disease in several ways. It facilitates oxygen supply to the heart muscle by promoting and improving collateral circulation. It actually reduces the heart's demand for oxygen by increasing that organ's efficiency. It improves lipometabolism, the body's use of fats. Regular systematic exercise helps lower the serum cholesterol level and reduces cholesterol buildup on the artery walls. It also speeds up the activity of the fibrinolytic system, helping break up clots of fibrin—a natural protein substance—into soluble fragments in the blood. This reduces the likelihood of clotting in the vessels. And equally important, exercise improves attitude. Not only does it direct attention away from disease, it gives a sense of health, control and optimism. All of these help prevent the recurrence of painful angina pectoris and other heart problems.

How Much Exercise for Coronary Patients?

A key factor in treating coronary disease with exercise is to determine the optimal amount and type of exercise. This is especially true for new patients. If the level of intensity is too low, the exercise will not improve heart efficiency. If it is too high, it may trigger angina or other symptoms. In fact, it may even endanger life. It's obviously important to choose exercises that are effective, yet safe.

Heart rate may be the best guide for determining the optimal level of exercise intensity. Heart rate, oxygen absorption and the capacity for physical exertion are related. And the heart rate seems to be the most accurate indicator of how much oxygen is absorbed by the heart muscle, as well as how much blood is circulating through the coronary artery. So, to determine the optimal level of intensity at which to exercise, you should determine your maximum heart rate. People who are young and healthy should do exercises that are strenuous enough to elevate their heart rate considerably.

In a study of physical exertion and heart efficiency, it was shown that consistent, long-term aerobic exercise did not improve heart efficiency when the heart rate stayed below 135 beats per minute. But when the same exercise was performed for the same amount of time at a higher intensity—heart rate of 150 or more—the subjects' heart performance significantly improved.

Another study reported that regular aerobic exercise did not increase the amount of oxygen absorbed when the heart rate was held below 130 beats per minute. Above this point, however, the amount of oxygen absorbed went up significantly. To have a positive impact on the heart and to prevent coronary disease, the young and healthy should regularly do exercises that raise their heart rates above 130.

For middle-aged or elderly people with coronary disease, the level of intensity should not be that high. If you are in this category, follow these guidelines:

1. The exercise should be intense enough to bring you near—but not over—the point where you suffer angina.

2. You shouldn't exceed 80 percent of your maximum physical exertion.

3. You should let your physician have the final say on a safe heart rate for you. The decision

Table 3
Heart Rates for Different Exercises

Types of Exercise	Heart Rates
Simplified *Tai Chi Chuan*	90 to 105
Fast walking	100 to 110
Swimming (100 meters at medium speed)	105 to 108
Table tennis	95 to 126
Jogging (medium distance)	120 to 140
Soccer, basketball	140 to 180
Physical labor (i.e., pushing a cart)	150 to 160
Martial arts	150 to 172
Running (medium to long distance)	180

Table 2
Maximum Heart Rates (MHR) for Coronary Patients during Healing Exercise

Age	Maximum Heart Rates *(200 minus age)*	Desired Heart Rates in Exercise *(80% of MHR)*
35	165	132
40	160	128
45	155	124
50	150	120
55	145	116
60	140	112
65	135	108
70	130	104

will be based largely on the results of your stress electrocardiogram.

In one study, doctors evaluated a small group of coronary patients for the relationship between their exercising heart rate and the occurrence of angina. Of 31 patients, 3 reported angina when the heart rate reached 108 beats per minute; 7 between 112 and 116; 8 between 120 and 124; and 13 between 128 and 138. Clearly, as their heart rates increased, their risk of having angina also increased.

For the second guideline, we can roughly estimate a patient's heart rate while at maximum physical exertion by subtracting age from 200. Multiply the resulting figure by 80 percent to get the ideal heart rate for the exercising coronary patient.

As shown in Table 2, coronary patients who are over 40 years of age should do exercises that will produce heart rates between 104 and 124. Some experts have suggested that the maximum heart rate during exercise by coronary patients should be 170 minus their age. Our experience indicates that patients won't develop angina if the heart rates are held below 110 during exercise.

Table 3 shows the expected heart rate for various exercises.

Precautions for Coronary Patients Doing Healing Exercise

Coronary patients who have angina pectoris and those recovering from heart attacks should consult their doctors about the amount and types of exercise they may do. If your doctor says you can do healing exercise, use intermittent training if your exercise consists mainly of leisurely walking, fast walking, jogging, bicycling and swimming. That is, exercise for 30 seconds and then rest for 60 seconds. Repeat this sequence 30 times. The entire session should last about 45 minutes. This method is suitable for patients with weak hearts and lungs.

Don't forget to allow sufficient warm-up before and cool-down exercises after each training session. Engaging in exercises of high intensity without warm-up activities invites angina. Stopping the exercise abruptly without first engaging in relaxation activities may also cause discomfort in the heart region.

Evaluate carefully your own unique condition before deciding on the type and intensity level of exercise. Never overstretch yourself to pursue a so-called maximum or optimal heart rate.

Before each exercise session take your pulse by counting for 10 seconds and multiplying by 6. Take your blood pressure then, too. Measure both again when you are exercising most vigorously and once more 2 minutes after you stop exercising. Use this information to monitor your body and to adjust the level of intensity of the exercise.

If you experience shortness of breath or dizziness during exercise, take longer breaks between intervals or perform rhythmic breathing exercises every now and then. If you feel extremely fatigued and experience chest congestion, shortness of breath, internal pressure or pain in the region of the heart, the upper left arm or the left side of the neck, you should terminate the exercise immediately and consult your physician.

Exercises That Help Heal Coronary Artery Disease

Depending on your age, your condition, your preferences and your surroundings, you can choose one or more of the following exercises recommended for people who want to protect their coronary arteries or who have arterial hardening.

Walking: Fast walking has a greater impact on the heart than leisurely walking. Fast walking —100 steps per minute—can raise the pulse to as high as 100 beats a minute or even higher. You should choose a pace and a step length that feels comfortable and allows you to breathe naturally. Don't be afraid to slow down if you get tired. You'll still be getting benefits. If walking is your only exercise, try to gradually aim for a total time of at least 45 minutes a day. You can break it into two sessions if you wish.

Slow jogging: Slow jogging is appropriate for people who are fit—who have regularly done other types of exercises. You can jog a short distance—50 to 200 yards—or a long distance —up to 2 miles. Monitor your heart rate and keep it under 120 beats per minute. Of course, if angina pain occurs following long-distance jogging, choose another exercise.

Pace-determined walking: This exercise has been found useful in clinics where people are recovering from arterial disease. But you can do it on your own. The first section of this exercise is better for people whose disease is more severe. As you gain strength, you can keep adding portions, until you are doing the whole course.

Start by walking on level ground for 3,000 yards. Complete the first 1,000 yards in 20 minutes and then rest for 5 minutes. Do the next 1,000 yards in 16 to 18 minutes followed by the same amount of rest. Allow yourself 20 minutes for the last 1,000 yards.

Next walk on level ground for 4,000 yards, about 2 miles. Complete half the distance in about 40 minutes, which includes a 5-minute break at the midway point. Then walk on a hill with a 30-degree to 45-degree slope for about 30 minutes. Take a 5-minute or 10-minute break and walk back the last 2,000 yards the same way you did before.

Swimming: If you have moderate physical strength and enjoy swimming, this could be the ideal exercise for you. According to one study of a group of middle-aged people, a 6-month swimming program produced a measurable improvement in their ability to absorb oxygen. The results were just as good as those obtained from fast walking. But don't swim so enthusiastically that you get overtired or chilled.

Ch'i Kung: Practice relaxation breathing or invigorating breathing using either the sitting or the lying-down position. (See the section beginning on page 44.) Don't try to breathe too deeply nor to hold your breath. *Ch'i Kung* is especially helpful for patients who are weak and nervous. You can expect that this exercise will improve the circulation in your extremities and produce warmth in the limbs. You may also get relief from dizziness, improve your mood and decrease the frequency and intensity of any anginal pain.

Comprehensive exercise program: This program includes a warmup, stretching, walking, slow jogging, relaxation exercises and simple therapeutic exercises such as ball passing, basketball shooting and badminton. These exercises are usually performed in a group in the afternoon. They generally last 30 to 60 minutes and are offered 2 or 3 times a week. The comprehensive lesson developed by the Sun Yat Sun Medical School in Canton is given in Set A on the opposing page.

Therapeutic gymnastics: Patients who are weak should stick to simple stretching and moving exercises. If anginal pain occurs when you're standing or exercising, start out with a lying-down position as a warmup. Gradually add sitting and standing postures. If pain occurs when you're at rest, try standing up and walking and doing your exercising while sitting and standing. If you're already fairly strong, start your exercises in a standing position. Whatever position you use, be sure to maintain an even pace and rhythm while working out, never overtaxing your strength, holding your breath or straining.

Recovering heart attack patients can also do therapeutic gymnastics. But these exercises shouldn't be started until 2 to 4 weeks after the event and not until the patient's condition has stabilized. A special program for heart attack patients is given in Set B on page 86.

Tai Chi Chuan: Composed of soft movements and easy relaxed postures, *Tai Chi* is excellent for heart patients who have high blood pressure. This exercise is widely recognized for its ability to lower blood pressure. *Tai Chi* also calms the nerves.

Set A: The Complete Set of Therapeutic Exercises for Patients with Coronary Artery Disease

1. Walk evenly and steadily for 1 to 1½ minutes.

2. Stand upright. As you take one step to the left, touch your fingers to your shoulders, then lift your arms straight over your head. Step back and lower your arms to your sides. Repeat, stepping right. Do this 8 times.

3. Stand upright. Step forward with your left foot as you bring your hands to your chest with palms down. Then reach forward as you exhale. Swing your arms around to the sides as you inhale, allowing your chest to expand. Repeat, stepping forward with your right foot. Do this 8 times.

4. Stand up with your feet apart and your hands on your hips. Turn your upper body first left and then right. Do 8 complete turns.

5. Stand upright. Take a step to the left as you bend your knees into a half squat. As you step and squat, touch your fingers to your shoulders. Return to the original position and do the exercise again stepping right. Repeat the sequence 8 to 12 times.

6. Stand upright. Step forward with the left foot as you lift your arms forward and over your head. Return to the original position. Repeat with the right foot. Do this sequence 8 times. Now take a 2-minute break.

7. While sitting with your hands on your hips, first bend your head forward then backward. Then turn it to the left as if looking over your shoulder, then to the right. Repeat 8 times.

8. Start by sitting with both hands on your thighs. Point your arms forward as if sleepwalking and lift one leg straight out. Stretch your arms to the sides. Return to starting position. Do the same with the other leg. Repeat 8 times.

9. As you sit with your hands on your hips, lean backward slightly and then forward slightly. Do this 8 times.

10. While sitting, form a circle with your arms in front of your chest. Then swing your arms across each other as if you were hugging yourself. Repeat 8 times.

11. As you sit with your hands on your knees, move your entire upper body in an easy circle. Make 4 circles.

12. Stand up from a sitting position as you lift your hands, with palms up, to shoulder level. Sit down and relax. Do this 6 to 8 times. Now take a 90-second break.

13. Stand and walk in place for about ½ minute.

14. Stand upright. Take one step forward with your left foot while making a circle with your arms, palms down, as if you were reaching around a tree. Then turn your body to the left as you extend your arms sideways, turning your

hands palm up. Return to the original position. Repeat with the right foot. Do this 8 times.

15. Standing with your feet apart, lean to the left as you touch your chest with your right hand. Stand straight, then repeat on the other side. Do this 8 times.

16. Stand with one foot directly in front of the other. Move your arms as if you were rowing a boat. Repeat 8 times.

17. While standing, step left as you lift your hands to touch your shoulders. Return to your original position. Repeat, stepping right. Do this 8 times.

18. Step forward with your left foot as you raise your left arm high. Step back, lowering your arm. Repeat with the right arm and leg. Do this 8 times.

19. Take a step forward with the left foot as you lift both arms up and over your head, reaching slightly behind and lifting your chin. Return to the original position and do the same with the right foot. This exercise may be repeated 6 to 8 times in a relaxed and easy manner.

20. Stand with your feet apart. Hold your arms to the sides with your elbows bent and your palms facing down. Rotate your upper body far enough so that on each swing, you can see the heel of your foot. You can do this exercise several times. The movement should be smooth and loose.

21. Walk steadily for 1 to 1½ minutes.

22. While standing, raise your arms to the sides as you lift your left foot with your knee bent. Return to the original position, then do the same thing using your right foot. Repeat 6 to 8 times, keeping your movements relaxed.

23. While standing, hunch your shoulders up and then relax them 6 to 8 times.

24. Standing with your hands on your hips, breathe in and out restfully 6 to 8 times.

25. Sit down and lightly massage your head, neck, face and chest with both palms for 3 to 5 minutes.

Set B: Healing Exercises for Patients Recovering from Heart Attacks*

Stage one: Begin these exercises no sooner than 2 weeks after your attack.

On the first day, do only the first three exercises. Add one exercise per day, doing each a total of no more than 5 times. After a week you can begin to add 1 or 2 repetitions per day until you are doing each exercise 10 times. If it feels comfortable, you can do 2 sessions a day. Do not move on to stage two for at least a week and make sure you get your doctor's permission.

1. Lie on your back and perform abdominal breathing quietly and naturally.

2. Lie on your back and flex and extend the toes.

3. Lie on your back and flex and extend the ankles.

4. While lying on your back, clench your fists and then let your hands relax.

5. As you lie on your back, raise your arms toward the ceiling and then lower them.

6. Lying on your back, contract your buttocks for a few seconds and then relax them.

---

*By modern Western medical standards, the progression of these exercises is too slow. After a heart attack uncomplicated by high blood pressure or other problems, doctors in the United States will usually have a patient sit up the first day and walk within 2 days after an exercise stress test. So don't be concerned if your doctor recommends more exercise than that described here. You should, of course, listen to your physician.

7. As you lie on your back, draw your legs up without taking your heels off the bed.

Stage two: Stage two lasts about 1 or 2 weeks. During this period, you can do the exercises in stage one and also begin sitting up, standing and walking. For the first 3 days, limit yourself to sitting up for no more than 30 minutes. On the next 3 days, you can sit up for a total of 60 minutes and stand up 3 times. For another 6 days, continue standing up only 3 times, but you can sit up for 90 minutes.

After this 10-day period, you can begin walking by your bed for 5-minute periods once a day. Gradually add a second 5-minute walk.

Stage three: Stage three lasts about 1 to 2 weeks also.

You're now allowed to walk beside your bed for 5 minutes at a time, 3 times a day. When you are completely accustomed to this, you may walk indoors for 50 yards the first day. The next day you can do 100 yards, then 200 the next, and 300 the day after. Stay at 300 yards once you have reached that level.

You can also perform the following exercises either sitting or standing. Start by doing each only once or twice.

1. Bend your arms at the elbows. Return them to a relaxed position.

2. Lift both arms forward as if you were sleepwalking, then lower them.

3. With your elbows bent, make circles with your arms to the sides.

4. Bend forward at the waist 40 degrees. Just let your arms hang. Then stand up straight again.

5. With your arms at your sides, bend your body gently from side to side. Breathe naturally.

6. Bend forward at the waist making a 90-degree angle and letting your arms swing free. Return to the original position.

7. Raise your heels. Lower them.

8. March in place.

If you are progressing satisfactorily, you may also practice walking up and down stairs. To start, walk only 4 stairs at a time. Add 4 more stairs every other day or every 3 days. Do not walk more than 40 stairs at a time.

Buerger's Disease

Thromboangitis obliterans (Buerger's disease) is a circulatory disorder that affects the smaller arteries and veins, and is marked by inflammation, deterioration of vessels and clotting. Why people get this disease is not fully known, but it is definitely associated with smoking. Western doctors believe that the inflammation of the blood vessels is the result of obstruction by a clot that has broken loose from the site where it was formed and caused an obstruction elsewhere. The disease prevents the tissues from getting an adequate supply of blood, oxygen and nutrients. As a result, gangrene may develop.

Traditional Chinese doctors attribute the condition to *ch'i* (energy) deficiency, blood and *ch'i* stagnation and inadequate nourishment. They also believe that the disease is related to overindulgence in heavily seasoned and greasy foods, excessively strong carnal desires and lack of sexual moderation.

The early symptoms of Buerger's disease, which occurs chiefly in young men, are feelings of cold and numbness in the extremities. The patient's legs turn pale and feel heavy and weak. At night the sufferer feels extreme pain. Sometimes the victim will limp. During the late stages of this disease, the patient can no longer feel anything in the affected limb because of tissue deterioration.

Because healing exercise strengthens muscles and blood vessels and facilitates circulation, it can help non-smokers prevent this disease. And in the early stages of the disease, therapeutic exercise can help control the affliction, especially when used in conjunction with other therapies such as acupuncture.

If the legs are affected, the most helpful exercises include walking on level ground for 30 minutes daily, broadcasting-drill type exercises (stretching and calisthenics), *Tai Chi Chuan* or canoeing.

Here are two special exercises for Buerger's disease:

1. While lying on your back in bed, raise your legs to form a 45-degree angle with your body. Hold this position for 1 or 2 minutes. Then dangle your legs over the edge of the bed for 2 to 5 minutes. Stretch your toes and move your feet at the same time. Rotate your feet at the ankles up and down, pointing in and pointing out, at least 10 times.

2. Lying on your back, lift your arms and legs into the air as shown in Fig. 54. Gently shake your limbs in this position for 1 to 2 minutes. Lower your limbs and rest, then do it again 5 or 6 times. This should be repeated at intervals of 3 to 5 times a day.

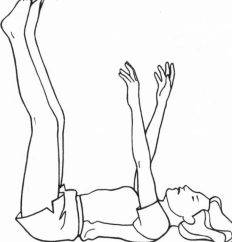

Figure 54. *Buerger's disease exercise helps circulation*

Can Purpura Be Prevented with Healing Exercise?

Purpura is a bleeding disease in which blood leeches into the skin, the subcutaneous tissues and the mucous membranes. It causes bruiselike purplish or reddish blotches. Unfortunately, thrombocytopenic purpura and allergic purpura —two common forms of the disease—cannot be treated by therapeutic exercise. In fact, serious cases call for bed rest.

Thrombocytopenic purpura can be identified by a deficiency of blood platelets and a prolonged clotting time. The blood platelet count often falls below 50,000 per cc. of blood. Allergic purpura, which frequently has a sudden onset, usually shows a normal platelet count and normal coagulation. Purplish spots may appear on the skin of the lower extremities as well as pale or red wheals. Severe abdominal pain, swollen and painful joints and blood with the stool or urine are also seen in cases of severe allergic purpura.

But the last type of purpura can be helped by exercise. It is a type which is frequently overlooked or misdiagnosed. Caused by blockage of blood in the veins—the result of prolonged sitting or standing—Chinese doctors describe it as being characterized by swollen and painful dark purple patches on the legs. Platelet count and coagulation time appear to be normal.

Physical exercises such as calisthenics and stretching, walking, *Tai Chi Chuan* and therapeutic gymnastics for the legs prevent this type of purpura—and they even cure it. The symptoms usually disappear a week or so after you begin exercising.

Warming Cold Hands and Cold Feet

In summer as well as winter, some people suffer from ice cold hands and feet. The condition may be caused by physical weakness and inadequate blood circulation in the capillaries. But in a majority of cases, the body's temperature regulation is malfunctioning.

In summer, people with this syndrome perspire so much that their hands and feet are constantly moist and chilly. In winter, their bodies—trying to conserve energy and keep their temperature up—constrict the smaller arteries and reduce the flow of blood to peripheral areas.

No matter what the season, people with this problem always feel cold in their hands and feet.

But this syndrome can be corrected through healing exercise. Ever since ancient times in China, people have used massage to relieve the condition. For example, in the classic text *Tsien Chin Fang* (The Thousand Prescriptions), the authors stated that "cold hands and cold feet can be relieved by the heat created by pounding." Massage can, indeed, improve peripheral blood circulation in the limbs. You can pound your arms and legs with a loose fist or clap them repeatedly with an open palm.

Coldness in the feet can be counteracted by rubbing the acupuncture point known as Bubbling Spring, located right in the middle of the sole of your foot. Do this right after getting up in the morning and just before bedtime. Continue rubbing until the foot becomes warm.

But to correct the underlying cause, you need to improve your overall physical strength and your body temperature-regulating mechanism. This can only be done through the systematic and persistent practice of a vigorous exercise.

The exercises *Ch'i Kung* and *Tai Chi Chuan* can also be used to treat this condition. According to one study, skin temperatures of both hands and feet—measured both objectively and subjectively by the feelings of the patients themselves—were higher during *Ch'i Kung* and *Tai Chi Chuan* practice. Just as for so many other afflictions, *Ch'i Kung* and *Tai Chi Chuan* once again offer relief.

CHAPTER FOUR

Breathe Easier with Exercise

康

Physicians in China have proven that exercise can benefit people with lung problems—even some of the most serious ones.

Doctors and physical fitness experts believe that both deep breathing exercises and other activities can help heal the lungs.

One measure of lung health is vital capacity —the maximum volume of air that can be exhaled after a full inhalation. For adult females, this amount is usually in the range of 2,500 to 3,000 milliliters. For males, it is 3,500 to 4,000 milliliters. But pleurisy patients, those with pneumonia, and those who are weak and underdeveloped may have vital capacities below the normal range. If vital capacity is too low—below 2,000 to 2,500 milliliters—the person may feel shortness of breath during exercise or physical labor.

Studies from both Europe and Japan have shown that deep breathing exercises can increase vital capacity. After 6 months of training, one group of young people increased their vital capacity by 300 to 400 milliliters. Other recent research suggests, however, that the results achieved by breathing exercise can be bettered. Deep breathing by itself doesn't do a thorough job of effectively stimulating the functioning of the lungs. Though it may help increase the vital capacity, it may not significantly improve respiration overall.

The most effective exercise for stimulating lung function, according to studies done in physical education, are exercises such as swimming, canoeing, basketball, jogging—exercises that demand the greatest performance from the whole respiratory system. A person who is playing basketball, for example, breathes 7 to 14 times the volume of air used while resting. During a strenuous track meet, air intake may be 15 to 20 times that of a rest period.

Other factors also play a role. Swimming and canoeing can help develop chest muscles, for instance. And while swimming, water pressure against the chest is believed to strengthen respiratory ability.

EDITOR'S NOTE: People who have breathing or lung problems should NOT take part in strenuous activities without consulting their doctor.

Lung and circulatory problems frequently go together and make vigorous exercise too risky. But *Tai Chi*, walking and slow jogging—simple, easy exercises that can be practiced year round, can be helpful even to those not able to do vigorous exercise.

Exercises such as swimming and canoeing can aid respiratory function, too, but care should be taken to avoid catching a cold or bronchitis—diseases to which lung patients have special susceptibility.

Preventing the Common Cold with Self-Massage

More than a thousand years ago, the Chinese discovered that cold-induced nasal congestion could be relieved by massaging both sides of the nose bridge. Later, acupuncturists learned that nasal congestion could also be eased by stimulating the *Yin Shen* (Welcome Fragrance) point located on both sides of the wings of the nose. These findings led to the discovery that colds could actually be prevented simply by massaging these points systematically. Here are techniques you can use to prevent the common cold:
• Rub both sides of the nose bridge with your opposing index fingers until the spot feels warm.
• Rub the *Feng Chih* (Windy Lake) point on both sides of the neck with your palms 30 to 60 times. (See Fig. 55.)
• Press on the *Yin Shen* points. *Yin Shen* is located near the most prominent part of the wings of the

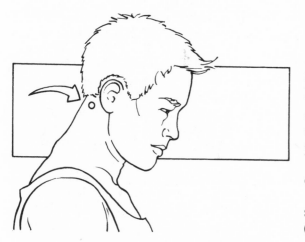

Figure 55. *Location of the right* Feng Chih *point*

nose as shown in Fig. 56. Lightly rub this area with the tip of your index finger 1 to 3 minutes.

• Rub the chest. Using the nipple as the center of a circle, massage the left chest with the right palm and vice versa. Make 10 to 20 circles on both sides.

How does self-massage help prevent colds? Probably by improving blood circulation and metabolism in the mucous membranes, increasing resistance to bacterial invasion.

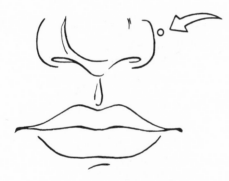

Figure 56. Yin Shen *acupuncture point*

Chronic Obstructive Pulmonary Disease

Chronic obstructive pulmonary disease refers to a family of lung disorders that gradually result in a decrease in lung function and an increase in difficulty breathing. The most common forms are emphysema and chronic bronchitis, both frequently accompanied by asthma.

Emphysema is characterized by a gradual destruction of the air sacs where carbon dioxide and oxygen are exchanged in the blood. As these small air sacs or alveoli degenerate, the surface area where oxygen and carbon dioxide exchange occurs shrinks, and the patient may suffer from a lack of oxygen.

Chronic bronchitis is a condition in which the air passages in the lungs—the bronchi—become inflamed. The inflammation results in mucus production and a narrowing of the airways, making both inhalation and exhalation difficult. A chronic bronchitis patient usually has a nagging cough, thick mucus and emphysemalike changes as well.

The term *asthma* refers to a reversible narrowing or spasm of the bronchial airways. This may be caused by allergic reactions, or simply by the inflammation already present in chronic bronchitis patients. Asthma frequently causes wheezing, coughing and mucus production.

Emphysema and Exercise

Many long-term sufferers of chronic bronchitis or bronchial asthma gradually develop symptoms of deterioration in their lung function, decrease in vital capacity and shortness of breath. When they are engaged in physical exercise or labor, they experience difficulty breathing.

Their problems are due to chronic irritation that causes the tissues of the bronchi and smaller tubes to become clogged with mucus. As the tubes become clogged and narrower and smaller, contraction of the bronchioles makes it even more difficult for air to pass through. At this stage, the patient begins to experience difficulty exhaling. As a result, pressure increases in the alveoli, the thin-walled air sacs where the exchange of oxygen and carbon dioxide takes place. The tissues become weak and less elastic. This leads to a breakdown in the lung structure, which makes exhaling increasingly difficult. Inflated unevenly with air, the lungs display constricted pulmonary emphysema.

Deterioration of the ability to breathe may be complicated by infectious diseases involving the respiratory tract such as pneumonia. Over a period of time, the heart function can also be adversely affected and eventually heart disease may follow. But this sorry scenario need not occur. Many victims of respiratory disease can be helped by healing exercise.

Exercises should be chosen by determining the level of health. Patients with pulmonary emphysema can be classified into four categories on the basis of their walking ability.

A. Patients who can walk on level ground as fast as the healthy of the same age and body build. They do not experience shortness of breath when they walk. However, they do not perform as well as their healthy counterparts at walking up and down stairs or over hills.

B. These patients can walk unhurriedly for 1 kilometer (⁶⁄₁₀ mile) without feeling breathless. But they cannot walk as fast as a healthy person on level ground.

C. This group of patients will experience shortness of breath after walking on a flat surface for just a few minutes.

D. The sickest patients feel breathless when doing simple tasks such as putting on clothes or talking with others.

The best time to begin a therapeutic program is when the disease is still in the early stages — patients in the first two categories. These patients can manage most day-to-day activities requiring little physical strain. But they may not be able to walk far and may experience shortness of breath while attempting to walk up and down stairs or walk over hills. When exercise is begun at this stage, patients can not only get better results than if they wait, but can also prevent the disease from worsening.

Patients whose physical condition falls into the last two categories may also benefit from exercise if they proceed in a cautious and systematic manner. Thus, healing exercise can benefit *all* emphysema patients as long as the disease is not complicated by acute infection or serious heart problems.

Treatment of emphysema should focus on preventing and controlling infection (mainly bronchitis and acute pneumonia), reducing inflammation, alleviating bronchiospasm, improving pulmonary function and enhancing the patient's overall health. Healing exercise does all these things.

In recent years, the emphasis on preventing and treating the so-called "three diseases" (the common cold, tracheitis and pulmonary emphysema) through exercise has been given special attention throughout China. The treatment worked. Effective techniques have been developed that can help pulmonary emphysema patients minimize the risks of catching colds and increase their walking endurance. Blood pressure and rate of breathing were both lowered in patients who consistently practiced healing exercise. And both vital capacity and the total volume of air passing through the lungs also increased even when patients were at rest. An overall improvement in patients' health had obviously occurred. There's no question but that patients with emphysema can be helped with physical exercise.

Exercises for Those with Emphysema

The best way of treating pulmonary emphysema with exercise emphasizes the body as a whole rather than merely focusing on improving the lungs. In other words, patients should not restrict themselves to breathing exercises alone, but should also do exercises that benefit the cardiovascular system and overall health. Improving the function of the other organs and the body as a whole will provide the most relief from emphysema symptoms. But lung patients who also have heart disease should consult their physician when embarking on an exercise program.

Therapeutic exercise for pulmonary emphysema can be divided into three categories:

1. Physical fitness exercises that aim at developing endurance, increasing strength and improving general health.

2. Breathing exercises that stress the importance of effective respiration, correct faulty habits and encourage muscle relaxation in breathing.

3. Massage, which is used especially to prevent common colds and lessen uncomfortable feelings in the chest.

Fitness Exercises for Emphysema Patients

The patient should walk between ¼ and ¾ mile daily. The starting pace may be as fast as is comfortable. The distance should be divided into three sections. At first walk slowly. For the mid-portion increase the speed slightly. The remaining distance is completed at a very slow speed.

Once a day, walking up and down stairs should be practiced. Patients who are relatively weak can start with the least demanding schedule. On the first day, you'll take 1 step up and 1 step down. On the second day, 2 steps up and 2 steps down. Each succeeding day adds another step until 24 steps up and 24 steps down have been reached. Once you've accomplished that goal, the amount of time should be gradually reduced until you can walk up and down the 24 steps within 18 to 20 seconds.

Patients who are in better shape may walk up and down stairs for 5 minutes each day. The height of all the steps mentioned should be between 6 and 8 inches. Walking and climbing up and down stairs should be part of the daily routine of emphysema patients.

Riding a stationary bicycle can also help to develop physical endurance. Use one with a tension-adjusting device. To begin, keep the tension at the lowest setting. The speed should be slow enough not to cause a strain.

Practice riding the bicycle for 5 to 7 minutes each day. After a while, you can ride 2 to 3 times daily. Later, practice periods can be increased to 15 to 20 minutes a day using the same degree of tension. Then gradually increase the tension level. Such gradual training is very beneficial in developing endurance.

Walking at intermittent speeds can help build strength. The patient should walk fast for the first 30 seconds and follow this with a 60-second period of very slow restful walking. Repeat 30 times. This exercise should be done 2 or 3 times a week. After 3 to 6 months, the exerciser will notice an increase in physical strength.

Calisthenics and stretching exercises are appropriate for patients who have adequate strength. But particularly helpful to the emphysema patient would be enrolling in a *Tai Chi*

Knocking at the Gate of Life

Chuan course. This relaxing dancelike exercise is excellent for relieving feelings of tension and anxiety. (See also the section beginning on page 33.)

For developing better lung function, basketball, swimming, hiking and jogging are great for new patients who are young and physically well equipped.

Breathing Exercises

Breathing exercises have a number of positive advantages for emphysema patients. First, they strengthen the muscles involved in breathing, especially the diaphragm. Having lost some of its expandability while under chronic stress, the diaphragm needs help regaining its mobility. However, a small improvement in the diaphragm can mean a big gain in breathing. If the diaphragm's expandability increases by 1 centimeter, studies show, lung capacity grows by 250 milliliters. About 2 centimeters of increase in the diaphragm can be achieved over time, with the corresponding exponential growth in lung capacity.

These exercises also help develop the habit of abdominal breathing, a method characterized

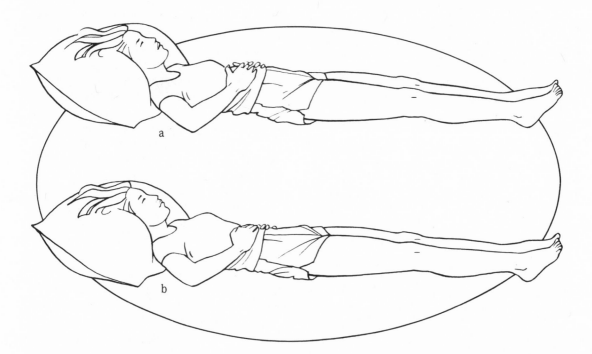

Figure 57. *Abdominal breathing*

by long, slow, deep inhalation and exhalation. Emphysema patients tend to breathe in a shallow rapid manner, relying primarily on chest muscles. This short, rapid respiration not only fails to allow sufficient passage of air through the lungs, but also tends to produce tension and fatigue in the chest muscles. Abdominal breathing helps eliminate these problems and facilitates the exchange of oxygen and carbon dioxide.

In addition, breathing exercises help reduce muscle tension and relax both the body and mind. Before starting relaxation exercises, patients should warm up with breathing exercises. A combination of the two types of exercise will produce the most effective relief of tension.

Last but not least, following breathing routines clears out phlegm, freeing the air passages from obstruction.

Breathing exercises for pulmonary emphysema patients emphasize abdominal breathing, which makes breathing out easier. Abdominal breathing depends on contraction between the abdominal muscles and the diaphragm. During inhalation, the diaphragm expands and moves downward, creating a pressure that forces the abdominal cavity to rise and the chest cavity to enlarge. The opposite effects occur during exhalation. The diaphragm moves upward to the original position and the abdomen falls.

The best position for learning how to do abdominal breathing is lying on the back. Place both of your hands on the abdomen. Then consciously breathe in and out slowly and deeply in a relaxed manner. As you inhale, you'll feel the abdomen rise. It will fall as you exhale. (See Fig. 57.)

Abdominal breathing can be mixed in with other kinds of exercises. It can also be performed using the methods of *Ch'i Kung*, especially the *Ch'iang Chuang Kung* (invigorating breathing technique). (See page 46.) Abdominal breathing should be practiced 2 or 3 times a day for sessions of 10 to 20 minutes. This training can help develop new breathing habits.

Here are some specific exercises particularly designed to help develop the ability to breathe out:

• This is a string-blowing exercise. Hang a string about 18 inches from your face. Exhale strongly to make the string blow in the wind. As you get better at this, you can move the string (or yourself) farther and farther away. (See Fig. 58.)

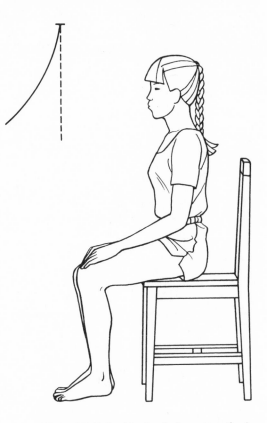

Figure 58. *String blowing for lung strengthening*

• With a straw, blow bubbles through water. Try to make bubbles for as long as possible. Try to make the bubbling last a little longer each day. (See Fig. 59.)

• Stand with your hands resting lightly on your hips. Breathe deeply, letting the exhalation take more than twice the amount of time required for inhalation. Breathe the air in through the nose, but breathe out through the mouth with the lips formed into a whistling shape. Let the air come out through the opening between upper and lower teeth or through the pursed lips. Remember to use abdominal breathing.

• Stand as in Fig. 60a with your hands against the sides of your waist as you inhale in through your nose. While exhaling out through your

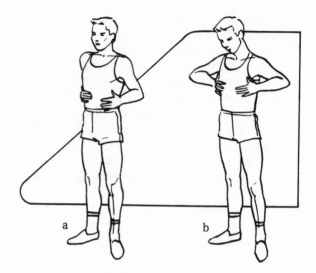

a   b

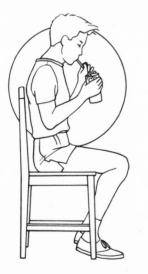

Figure 59. *Blowing bubbles for better breathing*

mouth, press your hands against the sides of your chest to aid in expelling the air. (See Fig. 60b.)

• Stand with your arms spread as in Fig. 60c while you inhale through your nose. While exhaling through your nose, squeeze your forearms against the upper abdomen to help the air come out. (See Fig. 60d.)

• Stand with your feet a shoulder width apart, your arms hanging loosely. (See Fig. 60e.) Breathe in deeply while lifting your head slightly upward. Then breathe out deeply while squatting down with both hands pressing firmly against the abdomen. (See Fig. 60f.)

• Sit down on a stool. Lace your fingers behind your neck. Slowly rotate your upper body from the waist. This exercise is designed to strengthen the joints between your ribs and vertebrae so that you can breathe more slowly and deeply.

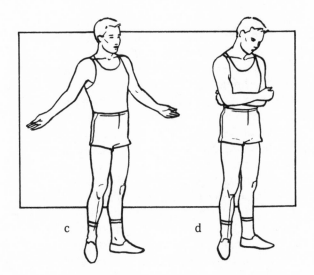
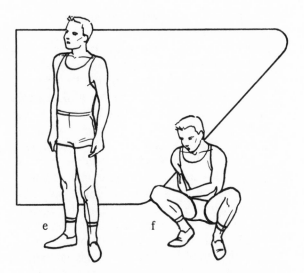

Figure 60. *Exercise to strengthen breathing*

The movement should be slow and steady. Reduce the speed if you feel dizzy.

These exhalation exercises should be practiced 2 times a day for 5 to 10 minutes. To avoid lightheadedness, limit the number of repetitions in each series to a comfortable level.

To achieve the best results from these healing exercises designed for pulmonary emphysema patients, they should be performed only after the inflammation in the respiratory tract is under control. And they should be practiced with regularity and persistence. Their ultimate purpose is to help the patient develop the habit of breathing abdominally all the time.

Massaging the Chest

Chest massage can be used to treat pulmonary emphysema, chronic bronchial asthma and cases in which the lungs are weak and susceptible to infection. It also has definite value in preventing the common cold. Chest massage is usually performed before breathing exercises. If postural drainage is necessary, this should be done before the massage.

Often chest massage can be performed by the patient. But if symptoms are pronounced and the patient is weak, the massage should be done by a medical professional.

There are several effective techniques for chest massage. One is the so-called vibration method. Sit in a straight-backed chair and wrap your arms around your chest as if you were hugging yourself. Your hands should be 1 or 2 inches under your arms. Now, creating a vibrationlike effect, rub your hands up and down your sides. The motion should be light and swift but with some force. Continue this massage for several minutes.

Another effective technique is clapping yourself on the chest. With your hand shaped as if you were going to applaud, clap the opposite side of your chest. Work down the outside, across the lower chest, up the front and finish under the collar bone. Repeat this sequence 3 to 5 times, then do the other side of the chest with your other hand. If a professional performs this massage, both sides can be done simultaneously.

Last but not least is the rubbing massage. Performed with an open palm, the rub should be light and should move circularly around the nipple. Rubbing as you go, 10 or 20 circles should be enough. All these methods aid breathing, relax chest muscles and help get rid of phlegm. Massage may be done 2, 3 or more times a day.

Elderly Bronchitis Patients Can Be Helped by Healing Exercise

Many older patients who have chronic bronchitis also have some degree of emphysema. They, too, can be helped by therapeutic exercise. Even if bronchitis patients have no trace of pulmonary emphysema, they should practice healing exercise to improve their overall fitness. It will better their lung function, prevent the common cold and help avoid acute attacks of tracheitis.

By combining medication with healing exercise, Chinese doctors in recent years have made significant progress in preventing chronic bronchitis. And patients who persistently practiced their exercises over a long period of time caught fewer colds. They also improved their lung capacity, their ability to take in oxygen and the strength of their diaphragms. Shortness of breath and chest discomfort were relieved.

The therapeutic exercises for treating chronic bronchitis in the elderly are basically the same as those used to treat pulmonary emphysema, including abdominal breathing exercises. But they also include a massage for preventing colds, cold water tolerance training and physical fitness exercises. The common cold prevention massage is described starting on page 92.

Chinese doctors have found that cold water tolerance training can help prevent bronchitis attacks and colds as well as increase tolerance to cold temperatures. Starting in the summer, the patient should begin washing the face with cold water, making sure not to neglect the nose. This washing should be repeated every morning. When the weather is warm, the patient may also rub cold water over the chest, or even over the whole body.

If you have chronic bronchitis but have sufficient strength, rapid walking, walking up and down stairs, jogging, hiking, *Tai Chi Chuan* and *Kuang Po Tsao*—the Chinese morning music drill or any simple calisthenic program—can be beneficial. You should try to exercise outdoors and get plenty of fresh air.

If you have a lot of phlegm, proper posture achieved with the help of exercise therapy can be of assistance in getting rid of it. Chest massage techniques such as those described starting on page 99 can also help. Physical therapists can also help you get rid of phlegm. First you should lie on your side with a firm pillow under your lower chest so that your body arches over it. Then while your chest is being massaged, have someone tap on your back to help loosen the phlegm and allow it to be expelled as you cough. This process will take 5 or 10 minutes.

Exercise and Bronchial Asthma

Many asthma patients wonder if healing exercise can help relieve a disease as hard to treat as bronchial asthma.

Well, let us examine the actual healing results of therapeutic exercise. Though generally speaking it may not be easy to treat bronchial asthma, with proper exercise it is possible to decrease the frequency of attacks and alleviate symptoms when they do occur. Young asthma patients were able to significantly improve the effectiveness of their breathing as well as their overall health by practicing healing exercise. Although they still had asthma attacks, they were far rarer. In a study done outside China, doctors reported that 70 percent of patients who did healing exercise have decreased asthma symptoms. Performing special breathing exercises prior to or at the beginning of the asthmatic attack can also prevent it from getting worse.

Here's how healing exercise can help asthma sufferers. First of all, the respiratory function, chest muscles and diaphragm of asthma patients tend not to be in good condition. Vital capacity is usually limited, lungs may have deteriorated and there is a tendency toward emphysema. But healing exercise can strengthen respiratory muscles and improve oxygen-carbon dioxide exchange. The possibility of developing emphysema is then greatly reduced.

Healing exercise can also reduce the incidence of bronchial spasms and improve blood circulation in the lungs. The mucus inside the bronchioles becomes thinner and easier to expel. Asthma symptoms are relieved.

Moreover, therapeutic exercise teaches a new breathing technique that prolongs exhalation. This breathing method can help reduce the duration of the asthma attack if it is performed before and right after the start of the attack.

Therapeutic exercises for bronchial asthma patients include pronunciation breathing exercises, corrective breathing, relaxation exercises, *Ch'i Kung* and massage.

Pronouncing words during exhalation conditions a new way of breathing by associating breathing with sound. This exercise can be done either while sitting or standing. While exhaling, pronounce the syllables *wu, e* and *ah.* When beginning this exercise, each syllable should be held only 5 or 6 seconds. But after practicing for a while, the patient may gradually increase the duration to 30 or 40 seconds. Breaks are permitted. You shouldn't become fatigued.

The corrective breathing methods are the same as those for pulmonary emphysema. The aim is to develop the habit of breathing with the abdomen and strengthen the process of exhaling.

The following relaxation exercises can help ease tense shoulder and torso muscles:

1. Standing with your arms at your sides, rotate your body to the side, letting the shoulders turn naturally. Do this 10 times. You can also turn your shoulders back and forth, concentrating on letting the shoulder joints relax completely.

2. While sitting, bend your arms into a circle in front of you. Let your shoulder joints relax completely. Swing the circle to the left then to the right about 10 times.

Massage can help relieve discomfort in the chest and back region. Patients themselves can massage the muscles that cover their ribs. Push and rub the chest area, and tap the back. This can be done by bending over and beating on the back with a loose fist. There is no limitation on how many times you may do this, as long as it feels comfortable.

Ch'i Kung—Ch'iang Chuang Kung (invigorative breathing) and *Fang Sung Kung* (relaxation breathing)—are good for patients with bronchial asthma. They are described starting on page 44. Sessions of 20 to 30 minutes 1 or 2 times a day will be beneficial.

The best fitness exercise for asthma patients is swimming. According to scientific studies, the incidence of bronchial spasm is lowered in swimmers. Patients with allergic rhinitis or recurrent ear infection should not dive or swim under the water, however.

Games that take from 1 to 2 minutes of playing time such as table tennis, badminton or shooting a basketball are also good for asthmatics. According to studies, these exercises help reduce the chance of obstruction in the respiratory tract. The worse the condition appears prior to practice, the greater the degree of improvement in clearing the respiratory tract after 1 to 2 minutes of exercise.

During exercise, bronchial asthma patients should use these rules as a guide. Healing exercise should only be practiced when the patient is free of asthma attack or when the attack is very mild. If asthma attacks recur frequently and the patient is not making gains in fitness, exercise should be discontinued.

Exercise time shouldn't exceed 30 to 40 minutes divided into 3 or 4 sessions. For example, 20 minutes should be devoted to *Ch'i Kung*, 3 to 5 minutes to self-massage, 3 to 5 minutes to pronounciation exercises with rest periods, and 1 or 2 minutes each to physical fitness and relaxation exercises. One or two sets of abdominal breathing exercises may also be included.

AUTHOR'S NOTE: Asthmatic patients should not exercise rigorously for more than 5 minutes at a time unless their condition is under good control. More exercising might aggravate the condition. But brief strenuous exercises lasting 1 to 2 minutes help reduce obstruction in the respiratory tract.

Before exercising, blow your nose to clear out mucus. If you experience chest discomfort or shortness of breath during practice, stop exercising and rest.

Exercises to Help Silicosis Patients

Silicosis is a common form of lung disease frequently found in miners and metal and foundry workers. It is caused by inhaling silica. The particles irritate lung tissues, impairing not only breathing but also general health. The patient becomes more susceptible to tuberculosis.

As part of a comprehensive program for the treatment of silicosis, therapeutic exercise can contribute to improved breathing and health. Symptoms such as coughing, panting and chest pain are lessened, and the patient's ability to use oxygen and take in and expel air get better.

Therapeutic exercises for silicosis patients consist mainly of breathing exercises, *Tai Chi Chuan*, calisthenics and similar routines.

However, breathing exercises should be avoided if the patient has active tuberculosis, is spitting blood or has heart problems.

Breathing exercises are intended to increase the diameter of the diaphragm and to extend the time spent exhaling. In addition to abdominal breathing, useful breathing exercises include those that call for the application of pressure to the abdomen or lower chest. For details, see the list of healing exercises for pulmonary emphysema starting on page 95.

Silicosis patients can also choose to do relaxation exercises and a combination of physical and breathing exercises such as the follow-ing sequence:

Sit on the side of a bed or a chair with your buttocks near the edge of the seat. Stretch both feet out in front of you and rest your palms on your abdomen. (See Fig. 61a.) Breathe in deeply. Bend the upper part of your body until your head is lower than your knees as you simul-taneously press both hands against the abdomen to help move the diaphragm upward, exhaling as fully as possible. (See Fig. 61b.)

Then relax both hands, raise your head and stretch your neck to the front while inhaling deeply as you slowly lift your body to the original position. By the time you're sitting up, you will have finished inhaling. Repeat this 7 to 14 times. Finally, stand and march in place for 1 or 2 minutes. Then do 7 or 8 full squats to complete this exercise.

Here's an excellent standing exercise. With your feet a shoulder width or a bit wider apart, bend your knees just slightly while keeping your back straight. Hold your chin up slightly and naturally, relax both your shoulders and waist and lift your arms with palms up. (See Fig. 62.) Breathe in lightly and out heavily. The time spent

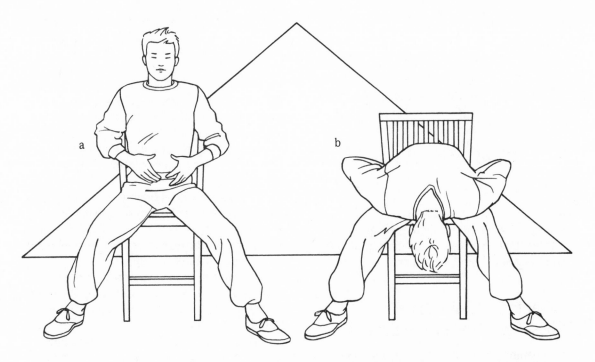

Figure 61. *Bellows technique to improve breathing*

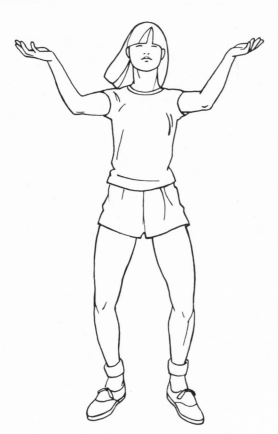

Figure 62. *A standing breathing posture*

inhaling is short. The exhale is long. Make your breathing natural and without the slightest effort. The breathing exercises for patients of pulmonary emphysema are good for you, too.

What to Do If You Have Chest Pain While Exercising

It sometimes happens that patients with serious respiratory problems experience chest pain dur-ing physical activities. The symptoms may in-clude pain that intensifies with conversation, breathing or coughing. A "crushing" type pain may also occur at times. But when you consult a doctor, no swelling, bruiselike hemorrhages or fractures are found. Nor do X-ray examinations reveal any abnormalities.

There are several possible causes of the pain. You might not have warmed up sufficiently, jumping into physically demanding exercise without adequate preparatory work. You may have neglected your deep breathing during your workout, and been breathing in and out without rhythm. The rate of your breathing may have been so rapid you weren't able to get enough oxygen. Your respiratory muscles may have been too tense for too long.

Or you may have started with a body that was overtaxed and weak. And you might not have participated in any form of exercise for a long time.

But what should you do? If the pain seems serious, of course you should see a doctor. If there is a possibility you injured yourself, you might need an X-ray. But if the results are nega-tive—if nothing is seriously wrong—there are some simple techniques that may relieve your chest pain.

Try taking a deep breath and holding it as you knock on your chest from top to bottom with a loose fist. Then breathe out slowly. Repeat this several times. The respiratory muscles will relax and the pain will be assuaged.

Or you can have another person pound the sides and back of your chest from top to bottom with a loose fist. Repeat this several times or until the pain stops.

Another tactic is to take several deep breaths and then press with your hand on the painful spot. The pain will usually go away. If someone else is doing this, have the person place one hand on the painful spot and the other opposite it on the back. The palms can then massage and press from both sides.

As simple a thing as lying down and rolling around in bed may also do the trick and relieve your pain.

Healing Pleurisy

Pleurisy is any condition that makes breathing painful. Usually, however, the condition that is referred to as pleurisy is caused by a viral infection, and this section refers to that type of pleurisy.

Patients recovering from pleurisy can help prevent pleural layers from adhering to each other—the problem that generally causes the pain—and improve their overall health with healing exercise.

Both wet and dry pleurisy can be helped by exercise. Dry pleurisy is characterized by a condition in which the surface of the pleura, the linings around the lungs, is soaked with fibrin, a protein from the blood. When the amount of fibrin becomes excessive, the parietal layer that lines the chest cavity and the visceral layer that covers the surface of the lung may stick to each other, causing chest pain during breathing. Other symptoms are cough and fever.

Dry pleurisy patients in the recovery stage may cautiously do breathing exercises. For the first few days, the patient should only do passive breathing exercises that don't involve movement of the limbs. Later, active breathing exercises accompanied by limb movements can be added. (Complete instructions start below on this page.) And gradually other exercises such as leisurely walking should be undertaken.

The other kind of pleurisy—pleurisy with effusion—is characterized by an accumulation of fluid, containing a great amount of fibrin, in the pleural cavity. The fibrin solidifies into fibers that cause the pleural layers to stick together and restrict the expansion of the lungs.

During recovery, patients can do a light amount of healing exercise once their temperature is almost normal, fluid is no longer secreted or is greatly reduced and the inflammation is under control. At this stage the patient can do simple exercises involving moving the limbs while lying flat or while lying down on one side. However, the patient should proceed to deep breathing exercises cautiously.

After further improvements in their health, patients may practice therapeutic exercise both while sitting and standing. Special attention should then be given to breathing exercises designed to strengthen respiration in the lower chest region. One of these would be placing both hands on the top of the head or lifting them over the head while concentrating on breathing in. Lower hands on the exhale. Another good exercise involves bending to the side with the opposite arm raised while inhaling. Straighten up again on the exhale and then repeat on the other side. Since many patients of pleurisy also suffer from tuberculosis, it is wise to adhere to the guidelines for therapeutic exercises for TB patients. And don't become overtired.

Set One: Pleurisy Exercises

1. While resting on your back, place both hands on your chest and experience relaxed chest breathing.

2. In the same position, rest both hands on your abdomen and breathe abdominally. (See also page 96.)

3. As you lie on your back with your hands by your sides, inhale while raising one hand at a time up and then back over your head. Exhale as you bring each hand to its original position.

4. Stretch your arms to the sides to form a cross and breathe in. Return to the original position while breathing out.

5. On your back, reach both your hands for heaven while inhaling. Breathe out while lowering your hands to your sides.

6. In a sitting position with your arms hanging at your sides, stretch each arm, in turn, straight out in front of you while inhaling. Breathe out while returning the arm to the original position.

7. In a sitting position, raise one arm in the air and bend to the other side while inhaling. Return to the original position while breathing out. Repeat with the other arm.

8. Sit down with your back straight. Lift both hands toward the sky as you breathe in. Return to the original position while breathing out.

9. While standing, lift both hands and place them on the back of the head as you breathe in. Return to the original position while breathing out.

10. Stand with both hands grasping a broomsticklike rod* in front of you. Lift the rod to chest level while breathing in. Return to the original position while breathing out.

11. Do a squat with a chair or exercise bar for support. Exhale as you squat, inhale as you rise.

12. Standing with both hands on your waist, lift one arm over your head and bend to the opposite side, breathing in. Return to the original position while breathing out. Repeat with the other arm.

*In China, exercise rods of this shape are in general use.

13. Breathe in while leaning backward with your arms in the air. Return to the original position while breathing out.

14. Hold a broomsticklike rod level to the ground in both hands behind your back. Bring the rod to shoulder level as you bend forward and tilt to one side and breathe in. Return to the original position while breathing out. Repeat while bending to the other side.

15. While standing, hold a broomsticklike rod in both hands across your thighs. Lift it directly over your head as you breathe in and bend to one side. Return to the original position while breathing out. Repeat, bending to the other side.

Set Two: Pleurisy Exercises

In the early stages of recovery, you should practice *Ch'i Kung* with emphasis on *Ch'iang Chuang* (invigorating breathing technique) while lying down. (See page 46.) This exercise should be done for 10 to 20 minutes, 2 or 3 times a day.

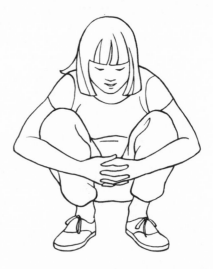

Figure 63. *Squatting exercise for deep breathing*

After your health improves, you may practice the same exercises either in a sitting or standing position. Then you may also try the following exercises:

1. Lift both arms up above your head while breathing in deeply. Then squat down with your arms around your knees while breathing out deeply. (See Fig. 63.) Repeat this 10 to 20 times.

2. Lift both arms up with palms facing out. While bending the upper body slightly to the front, perform deep breathing 7 or 8 times. (See Fig. 64.)

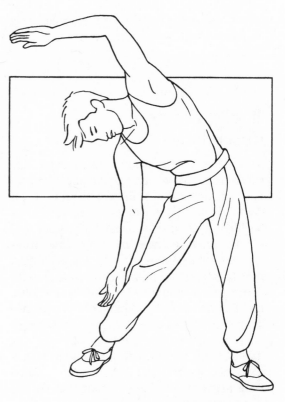

Figure 65. *The third set of* Pa Tuan Chin

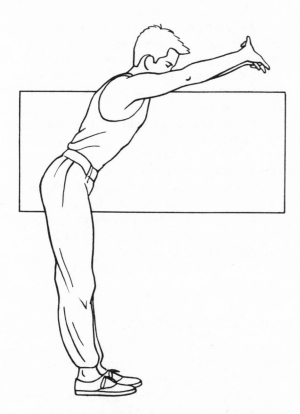

Figure 64. *Standing exercise for deep breathing*

3. With both hands above your head, bend the upper body to the left and then to the right 2 to 3 times. Stop bending and, with your hands still in the air, breathe in and out deeply 3 to 5 times. Repeat this exercise 3 times.

4. Perform the third set of the *Pa Tuan Chin* (Eight Sets of Embroidery on page 24) 2 to 3 times. This set involves lifting one hand over the head while lowering the other. (See Fig. 65.) While each hand is up, breathe in and out deeply 3 to 5 times. Repeat the entire sequence 3 times.

5. Squat down and up several times. This exercise should be followed by taking a stroll outdoors.

Treating TB with Healing Exercise

Until about 40 years ago, the treatment of tuberculosis relied heavily on rest therapy. Although this form of therapy is still somewhat useful, it doesn't help restore stamina, improve mental health or normalize the metabolic process.

But since the development of effective drugs to combat tuberculosis, medical practitioners have been able to combine therapeutic exercise with medication to treat the disease. In clinics, hospitals and schools in China, healing exercise has had positive effects on TB. Many young people who once suffered from pulmonary tuberculosis have regained their health and vitality with a combination of exercise and medication. Gains were made in the ability to maintain normal body temperature, in appetite, in body weight and in resistance to colds.

Experimental studies conducted in China positively prove TB patients can safely engage in healing exercises. And with regular practice, they can regain their health.

Medically speaking, the benefits of therapeutic exercise for tuberculosis patients include better performance by both heart and lungs, reduced risk of inadequate oxygen, improved metabolism and increased immunity. And aided by proper medical and nutritional treatment, therapeutic exercise can speed up recovery.

The right exercises can also help the body fight viruses and inhibit the spread of bacteria. Clinical experience confirms that symptoms such as fever and night sweats have been relieved in some cases and even eliminated by limited outdoor exercise. But whenever regular outdoor exercise was interrupted, the same symptoms reappeared. Resumption of the exercises cleared up the symptoms once again.

Doctors report that patients who suffer from the following two types of pulmonary tuberculosis will benefit the most from healing exercise:

1. Patients who have apparently recovered from the infiltration stage of tuberculosis may, depending on their physical condition, participate in exercise of medium to high levels of intensity.

2. Patients who are in the very early stage of the disease and are not experiencing symptoms may participate in less intense forms of exercise if their blood tests do not show any subsequent increase in white cells or reduction of lymphocytes.

Some TB patients should refrain from exercise. These include:

1. Victims of any type of pulmonary tuberculosis who are not yet in recovery.

2. Patients who feel extremely weak and who have lost over one-quarter of their body weight.

3. Patients who are spitting blood, who have lymph disease or tubercular infections in the kidneys, intestines or peritoneum.

4. Patients whose daytime temperature rises above 100°F.

Exercise for TB Patients

Healing exercises suitable for patients of pulmonary tuberculosis include gymnastics, *Tai Chi Chuan, Ch'i Kung*, walking and simple sports. Depending on their condition, patients should choose exercises of high, medium or low intensity.

Gymnastic exercise should be performed

early in the morning. Patients capable of high- and medium-level workouts may complete the whole set of the *Kuang Po Tsao* (music drill*), but the middle group should do only half of the repetitions. The weakest group should perform only a few of the most simple exercises.

The low- and medium-intensity groups may practice the short form of *Tai Chi Chuan*. The strongest group may do *Tai Chi* with slightly increased intensity.

One clinic in Peking used *Tai Chi* for the treatment of tuberculosis with good results. The beginners practiced the short form 2 times a day for 20 minutes each session. Having mastered that, the patients then moved to the medium level—practicing the entire series for about 30 minutes. After 3 months, the patients felt better and were healthier.

The weakest group of pulmonary patients may walk on level ground for 10 to 20 minutes. To start, they may walk once a day or once every other day. Later, after building up their strength, they can increase to twice daily. The middle group can walk 20 to 30 minutes a day to start. The strongest may take walks of 30 to 45 minutes 1 or 2 times a day.

Ch'i Kung is good for TB patients. Both *Fang Sung Kung* (relaxation breathing) and *Ch'iang Chuang Kung* (invigorative breathing) can help. Generally speaking, the lying-down posture is preferred. The medium and high groups may also use the sitting posture. Inhalation and exhalation during these exercises should be normal —spontaneous and unforced. Two 20-minute sessions a day are ideal.

According to traditional Chinese medical theory, *Ch'i Kung* stimulates *Yuan Ch'i* (inner energy) and enables the patient to build up an energy reserve in his or her body. *Ch'i Kung* is, therefore, an effective technique for treating tuberculosis. It's widely used in hospitals and clinics in China with good results.

Badminton is the best sport for TB patients. Young patients may also practice the basic movements of volleyball and basketball such as passing and shooting, without playing an actual game. Sports can be performed once a day or every other day for 10 to 20 minutes at a time. Soccer is too vigorous for tuberculosis patients. But table tennis is good if done indoors and in clean air.

Because swimming places a heavy burden on the respiratory system, and because of TB patients' increased vulnerability to colds, this exercise should be avoided for at least a year after recovery. However, patients who have the infiltration type of TB, who appear to be physically fit and who have entered the recovery stage can swim on warm days for 10 to 20 minutes per session. Chinese doctors recommend that care should be taken not to get excessive amounts of sun, which might reactivate the disease.

Points to Keep in Mind

In good weather, it's better for TB patients to exercise outdoors in the fresh air. Polluted areas, of course, should be avoided. Clean air is a necessity when exercising indoors, too.

Also avoid exercises requiring excessive amounts of energy, such as walking for over 3 miles, swimming more than 800 yards, and biking farther than 10 miles.

---

*In China, there is a national broadcast of a morning exercise program in which many people join. A rough equivalent would be a 45-minute stretching and calisthenics workout set to music.

Do not perform deep breathing exercises until the disease has been brought under control. Done too early, deep breathing may cause coughing and chest pain. However, when the disease has entered the sclerotic stage, some form of this exercise may be helpful. During deep breathing exercises, respiration should be as natural and relaxed as possible. Don't hold your breath for a long time and make your muscles tense. Strenuous exercises that cause breath holding and muscle tensing such as weight lifting or exercises on the bar should be avoided.

Exercise for TB patients should not cause excessive fatigue. Chinese doctors recommend that the weakest patients do no more than a total of 20 to 30 minutes of exercise, divided into morning and afternoon sessions. The middle group may work out a total of 30 to 45 minutes, and the strongest may exercise up to an hour all told. Time spent doing *Ch'i Kung* need not be counted in these totals.

Some tiredness after exercise is normal for everyone, of course. But recovery should occur after a short rest. If, following exercise, the TB patient has an increase in heart rate (pulse over 110 times per minute), palpitations, excessive sweating or fatigue even after 10 hours of sleep, the exercise has clearly been too taxing. The patient should rest for a few days before beginning healing exercise again at a lower intensity.

CHAPTER FIVE

Improving Your Digestion with Exercise

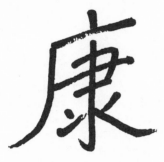

Sayings and lore in all cultures testify to the importance human beings accord to their digestive tracts. The Chinese, however, grant perhaps even more dignity and meaning to this system, and treat it with the appropriate respect. With that in mind, let's take a look at some of the successful ways the Chinese have discovered to heal their digestive tracts—from problems as common as constipation and hemorrhoids to such serious illnesses as ulcers and gallstones.

Curing Constipation

Changes in eating habits and bowel schedules are frequently cited as reasons for constipation. But actually the most common cause of habitual constipation is physical inactivity. And the best way to prevent or eliminate constipation is to exercise frequently, eat more vegetables, fruits and grains, and maintain a fixed bowel routine.

Therapeutic exercises, particularly those involving the abdomen and waist and those

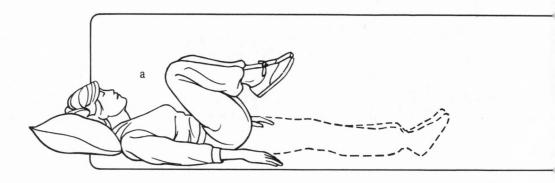

requiring jumping and deep breathing, can stimulate intestinal movement, strengthen the abdominal muscles and produce beneficial effects on the nervous system. The latter in itself helps prevent constipation.

People who suffer from habitual constipation can benefit the most from therapeutic gymnastics, exercise therapy, the *Ch'i Kung* breathing techniques and self-massage. (See the section starting on page 40.) The following gymnastic exercises are especially helpful.

Therapeutic gymnastics: To stimulate the abdominal region, it is recommended that the following four exercises be performed:

1. Leg bending: Lie on your back with your legs out straight. Bend your legs, raise them and draw them in to touch your abdomen. (See Fig. 66a.) Return to your original position. Repeat this 10 or more times.

2. Leg lifting: Lie on your back with your legs out straight. Lift both legs simultaneously without bending your knees and then slowly lower them, keeping your knees straight. (See Fig. 66b.) Repeat this 10 or more times.

3. Pretend peddling: Lying on your back, lift your legs into the air and pretend to peddle a bicycle. (See Fig. 66c.) Your movements should be relatively quick, rhythmical and smooth. Perform this exercise in 20- to 30-second bursts.

4. Sit-ups: Starting on your back with your arms stretched out over your head, do sit-ups, reaching all the way down to touch the tips of your toes. Do this 7 or 8 times. (See Fig. 67.) (If this is too difficult or hurts your back, you can do partial sit-ups with knees bent and arms at your side.)

Exercise therapy: The most effective exercises are walking, jogging and canoeing. The best time to walk is in the early morning. Right after getting up, go outdoors and walk at a fast pace for 30 minutes. If you are physically weak, you may take a leisurely walk for approximately 15 minutes after breakfast—if it's okay with your doctor. Afterward, drink a glass of water and then attempt to move your bowels. A regular outdoor walk of 1½ or 2 miles is also recommended anytime during the day.

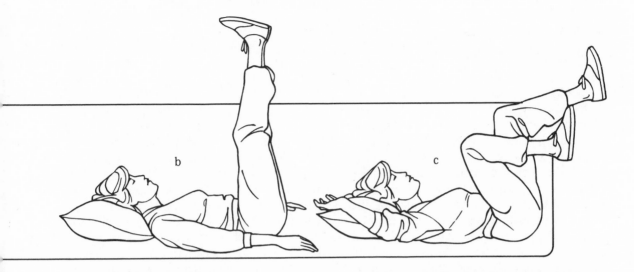

Figure 66. *Therapeutic gymnastics for the abdomen*

The vibrations produced by running and jumping also have a stimulating effect on the intestines and facilitate bowel movements. People who are physically fit may jog, play basketball and do similar exercises. The rowing motion in canoeing can also stimulate intestinal movement. For this reason, regular canoeing can help prevent or relieve constipation.

Water bath: Depending on your physical condition, you may rub your body with water, take a shower or simply go swimming. If you can stand it, use cold water which is more effective in stimulating the intestines. But if you find cold water intolerable, a warm water bath may be taken instead. The best time for a warm water bath is in the morning after exercise.

Ch'i Kung: The *Nei Yang Kung* (internally nourishing exercises) are recommended for people with constipation problems. You should perform these abdominal breathing exercises for 30 minutes or so in a lying-down position. (See page 49.) Do this 2 or 3 times a day.

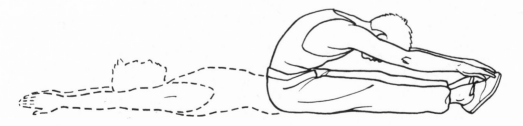

Figure 67. *Sit-up from a stretch*

Ch'i Kung works to prevent or treat constipation because it improves emotional states. It also works because it restores the proper balance between sympathetic nervous system inhibition and excitation vital to normal bowel functioning. And during deep abdominal breathing, the diaphragm moves up and down rhythmically massaging both the stomach and intestine. During abdominal breathing, the activity of the diaphragm is 3 to 4 times greater than normal. If someone were to put an ear to your abdomen, the results of *Ch'i Kung* would be clearly audible.

Massage: While lying flat on your back with your legs bent slightly and your knees supported by a pillow, perform self-massage by pushing and pressing down on the abdominal region with one hand on top of the other. Start the massage on the lower right side of the abdomen, then move up to the rib area. Continue in

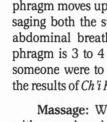

Figure 68. *Movement for massaging the abdomen*

a circular motion, moving to the left side, crossing over the navel and rubbing until the hands reach the lower left side of the abdomen. Rub and press against this area slowly but deeply before returning to the original position. The entire sequence will count as one circle. (See Fig. 68.) Do this 30 or 40 times. If you prefer, you may massage by the clock for, say, 10 minutes. After your abdominal massage is completed, sit down and lightly tap the sacrum area (the hard area in the small of your back). This massage may be performed 1 or 2 times a day. It is particularly good after therapeutic gymnastics or *Ch'i Kung*.

To enhance the treatment process, the constipated person should also pay careful attention to diet. Eat a lot of greens and fresh fruit and drink plenty of water. Add whole grains, bran, lentils and beans to your diet. A small amount of honey may be helpful, too.

Relieving Indigestion with Massage

When the digestive system is impaired, belching, nausea, vomiting, abdominal pain and gas will occur. Massaging the abdomen will alleviate these symptoms.

The use of massage as both a preventive and as a healing technique has a long history in Chinese medicine. For example, one ancient classic medical text says that "indigestion can be relieved by first massaging the abdomen with both hands and then walking a distance of one hundred steps." The same book mentions that "massaging the abdomen after a meal can aid the functioning of the spleen and prevent indigestion."

Studies have shown that massaging the abdominal region not only heightens the level of activity in the stomach and intestines but also promotes circulation in the abdominal cavity.*

Here is an indigestion relieving massage technique: rub the palm of your hand on your upper left abdomen. If this region is distended due to the presence of gas, perform the massage with a vibrating finger motion. Move to the lower right abdomen and massage in a circular motion around your navel, moving up from the bottom and from the right to the left. A small amount of pressure can be applied while you are rubbing. The session should last about 20 minutes. You may perform the massage yourself or have someone else do it for you.

Strengthening the Muscles of the Abdominal Wall

Many middle-aged individuals and young mothers have a slack abdominal wall. Their abdomens hang forward and down. Although some people have not yet reached the stage where their bellies are hanging down, they do have a slack abdominal wall. Their abdomens have become distended and large. Weak and loose abdominal muscles are responsible. And sometimes excessive fat deposited in the abdominal wall has aggravated the problem.

Although a slack abdominal wall is not in itself a disease, it can, if uncorrected, lead to other ailments. For example, individuals who

have a slack abdominal wall are likely to develop constipation. Their abdominal muscles are simply too weak to contract properly. The abdominal wall cannot exert sufficient pressure to move the bowel.

Another problem created by an out-of-shape abdomen is that the body is forced to readjust its center of gravity. To adapt to the distended abdomen, the lumbar vertebrae turn forward, creating strain on back muscles. This is why people who have slack abdominal walls are more likely to also suffer lumbago.

Loose abdominals also lead to problems with indigestion because the excessive fat stored in the area hampers blood circulation and impedes digestive functions.

To correct a slack abdominal wall, you can strengthen those muscles alone or do exercises that will improve your body as a whole. These are particularly important for people who are overweight because whole body exercises use up more energy and have a greater impact on cutting down the amount of fat storage.

Exercises to strengthen the abdomen range from simple to complex. Individuals who are physically weak should perform only simple ones. The gymnastics recommended for constipation (see page 112) are excellent for strengthening the abdomen. Exercises that involve holding a dumbbell or a sandbag may not be appropriate for the physically weak.

*Symptoms of indigestion may be caused by a multitude of physical disorders. If they are severe and persistent, you should consult your physician. In some cases, heart trouble has been mistaken for indigestion. If you experience lightheadedness, shortness of breath, weakness and sweating with your indigestion, consult a doctor.

Preventing Hemorrhoids

Hemorrhoids are a very common affliction. In China, one survey found that 60 percent of urban and 70 percent of rural residents suffered from hemorrhoids.

Why do so many people have this problem? Research has identified several factors that contribute to the prevalence of this condition.

Habitual constipation, poor eating habits and indulgence in foods with strong seasoning, cases of persistent diarrhea or dysentery, chronic stomach and intestine diseases, aging and a generally weakened body condition and slack muscles are some of the primary causes. A rise in the pressure of the portal veins, cirrhosis and an increase in the pressure in the abdomen caused by pregnancy or tumors, high blood pressure, arteriosclerosis or chronic inflammation of the rectum may also contribute, Chinese doctors believe. Perhaps the most important factor is simply that human beings walk on two feet instead of on all fours. Animals who walk on four feet do not get hemorrhoids. Their pelvic cavities do not have to support their abdominal organs.

To further understand this common condition, we must look at blood circulation. The return of venous blood to the heart relies on muscle contraction and the functioning of valves inside the veins. The valves make sure that the blood in the veins can flow only in the direction of the heart and never away from the heart. To prevent the flow of blood in the wrong direction, human beings are equipped with valves below the level of the heart. Unfortunately, the rectal veins are not equipped with valves because our evolutionary design intended our rectums to be on the same level as our hearts when we walked. Thus, the blood can back up in these vessels and pressure caused by gravity, strain or other factors can cause these veins to distend into hemorrhoids.

But hemorrhoids can be helped. The following nine exercises have healing benefits for hemorrhoid sufferers. People who have anal fissure or prolapse of the anus with acute inflammation should not engage in these exercises. Acute inflammation must be treated with medicine before proceeding with exercise. You can expect to see results in 3 months if you practice these exercises 1 to 3 times a day. If time is a problem, you may do exercises 1, 5 and 6 only. After the condition has been brought under control, you may practice the anal constriction exercises to speed recovery. These exercises should be

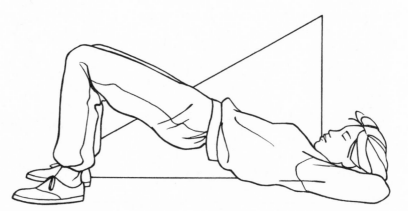

Figure 69. *Lying-down exercise for hemorrhoid healing*

practiced in a persistent manner with gradually increasing intensity to achieve maximum benefits.

1. Lie on your back in a relaxed position and cross one leg over the other, letting it rest there. Then press your inner thighs together while at the same time tightening—in China it is called lifting—your anus. Repeat this squeeze 10 to 30 times. As you become accustomed to this exercise, you may begin to combine it with breathing techniques, inhaling deeply as you squeeze and exhaling as you relax.

2. Lie on your back with your knees bent and your hands under your head. Raise your pelvis as shown in Fig. 69 while simultaneously lifting and constricting your anus. Then, lower your pelvis and relax the anus. After a while, start practicing constricting the anus during inhalation and relaxing it during exhalation. Work up to 8 repetitions.

3. Next, use a self-massage technique. Placing your hand so that *ch'i hai* (the Sea of *Ch'i* or energy), which is located directly below the navel, is in the center, rub your abdominal muscles. Rub first in a counterclockwise direction, 20 to 30 circles, and then reverse directions.

4. Lie on your back with your arms resting beside your body. Relax. Then without bending your elbows, raise your arms up, back and over your head as you breathe in deeply. Exhale as you bring your arms back to your sides. Repeat 5 or 6 times.

5. Sit on the floor with your legs crossed. Relax your entire body. With your legs still crossed, stand up, keeping your legs tightly against each other while constricting your anus. Keeping your legs crossed, sit down again and relax completely. Repeat 10 to 30 times.

6. Standing with your legs crossed, press your legs tightly against each other while constricting your anus; without uncrossing your legs,

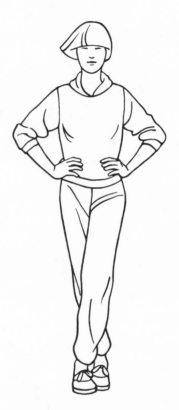

Figure 70. *Standing exercise that may help hemorrhoids*

relax your body as much as possible. (See Fig. 70.) Do this squeeze-and-relax sequence 20 to 50 times, depending on your physical condition.

7. Stand with your legs crossed, inhaling as you press your legs against each other, and tighten your anus. After a full inhalation, breathe out while knocking lightly against your abdomen with loose fists. Repeat the tightening and knocking sequence 20 to 40 times. The force of the "knock" should be increased gradually and cau-

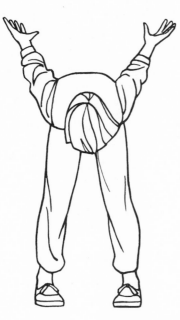

Figure 71. *Bowing with the arms back*

tiously. If you feel discomfort in your abdomen, reduce the intensity. This exercise should not be performed by pregnant or menstruating women.

8. Stand with your feet a shoulder width apart. Make loose fists and lift them to the sides of your chest at nipple level as you breathe in. Keep your elbows back, your chest open and your head up. As you exhale, bend gracefully forward into a deep bow with hands stretched backward and up and your palms open. (See Fig. 71.) Repeat this 5 or 6 times.

9. With your feet close together, stretch your arms over your head and rise up on your toes as you inhale deeply. Exhale as you return to your original position. Repeat 5 to 6 times.

Exercises to Help Prevent Rectal Prolapse

A prolapse of the anus takes place when the mucous membranes that line the rectum are displaced downward. The internal mucous membranes detach from the underlying wall and protrude from the anus.

Rectal prolapse may be caused by a number of factors. In young patients, the ligaments and muscles which make up the pelvic floor may not have developed enough to be able to give proper support to the rectum. Poor health in general, malnutrition or recurrent diarrhea can also contribute to this condition.

In elderly patients, rectal prolapse may be caused by a combination of poor health, slack muscles and ligaments, and gravity's pull on the stomach and intestines. Frequent childbirths in women who lack physical fitness can cause the muscles that support the rectum to become slack. A chronic cough or abdominal pressure from other sources can also cause a prolapse of the rectum. Having hemorrhoids, a slack sphincter muscle or a rectal fissure can also contribute to the creation of the problem.

According to traditional Chinese medicine, prolapse of the rectum may be symptomatic of a number of underlying conditions. Chinese doctors believe that the most important causes of rectal prolapse are deficiencies in internal energy and blood. In the elderly, a gradual diminution of blood and energy, coupled with extended illness, can lead to serious deficiencies. When energy and blood are in short supply, the body fails to absorb a sufficient amount of nutrients.

Chinese medicine recognizes a close connection between overall health and the condition of the perineum and the anus. Overall health can be improved through a conscious effort to keep the anus in good condition. Ancient medical specialists recommended frequent use of an exercise known as "closing the gate," in which the anus is constricted. Many Chinese martial arts also emphasize the exercise of "lifting" the anus as part of their training program.

Just like muscles in the arms and legs, the muscles that make up the pelvic floor can be strengthened by exercise. And these exercises are effective in preventing prolapse of the anus.

The same techniques designed for hemorrhoids can be used for treating prolapse of the anus. However, patients with anal prolapse should practice the exercises mainly in a lying-down position. Before starting any exercise, the patient should push any protruding portion of the rectum back into its original position. The exercise should proceed gradually and cautiously. If acute inflammation occurs, it should be treated before resuming an exercise schedule.

Self-Massage for Stomach and Intestinal Problems

Ulcers, irritable stomach, fallen stomach and habitual constipation can be treated by self-massage. The following are two massage techniques that have been found to be effective. You can choose between them on the basis of which feels better.

1. Kneading the abdomen: Before getting up in the morning and just before going to bed, you should knead and rub around the navel with one hand in the counterclockwise direction. Using one hand, make 30 to 100 circles. Apply some pressure when kneading, but don't hurt yourself. Then go clockwise with the other hand.

2. Pointed finger massage: Press down with your fingertips slowly but with some force at any spot on your abdomen. Press as deeply as possible without pain before releasing the fingers slowly. Press each spot deeply 3 to 5 times. Although one can start the pointed finger massage anywhere, it is preferable to begin at a spot on the upper abdomen. And it's best to follow a systematic pattern—moving around the edges and spiraling inward, for instance.

If done regularly, this pressing exercise will not only alleviate stomach and intestine-related diseases, but will also improve general health and encourage restful slumber.

Do not perform this exercise after a heavy meal, however. And refrain from doing it if there is acute inflammation, tumor, bleeding or high fever.

How long should you knead, point and press? Basically as long as you find comfortable. Many patients with chronic stomach and intestine diseases obtain excellent results by kneading the abdomen several hundred times.

Healing Stomach and Intestinal Ulcers

Ch'i Kung has proved to be a very effective technique in treating gastric and duodenal ulcers (ulcers in the stomach and upper part of the small intestine). In China, numerous studies have shown that practicing Ch'i Kung over an extended period of time relieved upper abdominal pain for many patients. X-rays taken after Ch'i Kung therapy showed that their ulcers had vanished. Their digestion returned to normal, their appetites improved and they gained weight. There was an overall improvement in their health.

Why is Ch'i Kung so effective in treating ulcers? The main reason is that the mental quietness and tranquility associated with the *Ch'i Kung* state has an inhibitory effect on cortical activity—active thought processes. Overexcitation of the cerebral cortex, a part of the brain, and the development of ulcers are closely related. Emotional states such as anxiety, nervousness or extreme excitability, linked to cortical over-activity, may also precipitate the onset of ulcers. But the relaxation and tranquility brought about by *Ch'i Kung* are effective antidotes for ulcers.

Nei Yang Kung and *Fang Sung Kung* (both the internally nourishing and the soothing techniques) are beneficial to ulcer patients. Practice these techniques by using either the lying-on-your-side or the sitting position on page 44. Do these exercises for 30-minute sessions, 2 or 3 times a day.

In addition to *Ch'i Kung*, ulcer patients may practice *Tai Chi Chuan* and abdominal massage. A proper balance between activity and relaxation should be maintained. If your condition is serious, you should postpone exercising until it has improved or stabilized. Strenuous exercises might cause severe pain or even result in bleeding or stomach perforation. Be careful.

Don't forget the tie between emotional states and ulcers. A spirit of optimism can speed up recovery. Anxiety and impatience may have an adverse effect on the treatment process.

How Physical Exercise Can Help Diabetes

One formerly diabetic patient in China who was successfully treated with exercise therapy described his treatment this way: "I always walked one thousand steps before each meal and two hundred steps after. I tried not to overeat and I cut down my sugar consumption.

"I was consistent in following my walking schedule before and after each meal. After six months, I noticed I'd lost a lot of weight and that my diabetes was a lot better. Eventually, I recovered completely."

The account given by this patient of the treatment of his diabetes through exercise is nothing new. In fact, Ch'ao Yuen Fan, a famous Chinese doctor of the Sui Dynasty, wrote in his medical classic *Chu Ping Yuan Hou Lun* (*On the Causes of Diseases*) that patients suffering from diabetes-related diseases should "first walk one hundred and twenty steps or more, not to exceed one thousand steps. Then after doing this, they should take their meal." Wang Shou, a famous doctor of the T'ang Dynasty, gave similar advice and suggested that exercise could also be used to *prevent* diabetes.

Physical exercise, diet, oral hypoglycemic agents and insulin therapy are the major approaches to the treatment of diabetes used by most specialists.

Clinical experience in China has demonstrated that therapeutic exercise is of indisputably great benefit to the diabetic. Exercise contributes to proper utilization of sugar by the body. In one group of diabetic patients tested, the level of sugar concentration in the blood fell significantly after only 30 minutes of therapeutic exercise. Because blood sugar levels dropped, symptoms such as sugar in the urine and frequent urination were also reduced.

The total volume of urine, usually abnormally large in diabetics, was reduced by up to a quart daily in this group of patients. These experiments and other experience in clinical settings have shown that healing exercise can help reduce insulin consumption, improve the ability to breathe, reduce the pain in the joints and relieve diabetes-related itching and constipation.

Healing exercise will be most effective for patients who have relatively mild diabetes. Exercises frequently recommended include *Ch'i Kung, Tai Chi Chuan* and leisurely walking.

From the breathing techniques of *Ch'i Kung*, choose *Nei Yang Kung* (see page 49) and practice twice a day for about 30 minutes each time in either the lying-down or the sitting position.

You should do *Tai Chi Chuan* once a day—either the simplified or the original version, depending on your condition.

Leisurely walking after a meal can increase your rate of metabolism. Studies have shown that metabolism can be increased 48 percent at a walking speed of only 2 miles an hour.

If you are in good shape, you may also go on hikes, canoe or take part in other such activities. These moderately demanding outdoor workouts can also be of great benefit to diabetics.

We suggest that no exercise other than a leisurely walk be undertaken immediately after breakfast. And if your diabetes is seriously incapacitating, you must refrain from exercise until it can be brought under control.

Before starting on any exercise regime, diabetics should consult with their physician, who will want to monitor blood sugar levels. As exercise levels increase, insulin or drug levels may decrease. If the proper adjustments are not made, blood sugar levels may drop too low.

Preventing Gallbladder Disease with Healing Exercise

Cholecystitis, an inflammation of the gallbladder, may occur by itself, but it is usually accompanied by cholelithiasis—gallstones. A chronically in-flamed gallbladder is one of the most frequent causes of digestive disorders. The patient often suffers from a bloated feeling, belching, constipation and the inability to digest fatty foods. After a heavy meal if you have gallbladder trouble, you may feel discomfort in your upper abdomen. Pains in the lower corner of your shoulder blade and in the right side of your waist, may occur often, particularly during standing exercise, bending or rising from a sitting position.

When the bile duct is obstructed, an acutely inflamed gallbladder will result and cause severe pain and jaundice. In some patients, this condition may be responsible for the onset of heart disease, Chinese doctors believe.

Inflamed gallbladders and gallstones are caused by sluggish bile. Thick bile may be associated with infection, defective bile ducts, a chronically inflamed liver, or metabolic imbalances. An infection may also be aggravated by the gallstones themselves.

Studies have shown that physical exercise can stimulate the liver to more than double the amount of bile it secretes. Regular and systematic healing exercise, especially breathing exercise, stimulates the organs in the abdominal cavity and facilitates the secretion of bile. By keeping the system flowing, exercise can be an effective means to prevent gallbladder problems. It is particularly useful to patients who are recovering from chronic liver inflammation.

Under certain conditions, exercise may not be appropriate. For example, in the case of repeated gallbladder infections coupled with other complications, surgical removal of the gallbladder may be the only recourse. Healing exercises are useful for treating gallbladder inflammation and stones when they have not reached the critical stage.

Based on your condition, you and your

doctor can choose from among the following exercises:

A. A leisurely daily walk of 30 minutes or so. In the beginning, your pace should be slow and easygoing. When you're better, you may increase your speed gradually.

B. Breathing exercises. The ones listed for silicosis patients in Chapter Four (see pages 102–104) are perfect.

C. *Tai Chi Chuan*. You can practice from 1 to 3 times a day.

D. The exercises recommended for hepatitis patients (see below).

Exercise and the Hepatitis Patient

As long as their livers are functioning normally, chronic hepatitis patients may do healing exercise. It can help improve their overall health, speed up their recovery and help them build up their physical strength. But patients should check with their own doctor before starting an exercise program.

Healing exercise will alleviate hepatitis-related problems such as jumpiness, insomnia and depression, Chinese physicians say. Another major healing factor is its promotion of blood circulation in the abdominal cavity and improvement of digestion. Healing exercises helpful to hepatitis patients include *Ch'i Kung*, massage and *Tai Chi Chuan*.

You should practice the *Nei Yang Kung* technique of *Ch'i Kung* (see page 49) in a lying-down or sitting position. If you use the prone posture, you should lie on the right side of your body to perform the abdominal breathing. Do this exercise for 20 to 30 minutes, 2 or 3 times a day.

Self-massage can be very helpful in facili-

tating circulation in and around the liver. While lying on your back, rub the area from your lower right chest to your upper right abdomen with your right palm from 100 to 200 times. Count each up-and-down stroke as 1 time. If you get tired, change hands. Do this massage once in the early morning and again just before bedtime.

In your *Tai Chi* workout, use the simplified version. Remember to keep your movements very slow and smooth. Breathe in and out abdominally unless it causes you discomfort.

Once a day or every other day you can take a slow walk or play ping pong or badminton for up to 20 minutes.

Should chronic hepatitis patients do abdomen strengthening exercises? This question is important because some patients felt discomfort around their livers after exercising.

Strenuous exercises that may stress and overwork the abdominal muscles, causing discomfort in the liver area, such as sit-ups and on-the-back peddling indeed are not appropriate for recovering hepatitis patients. They should not do exercises that actively involve the abdomen. Less demanding exercises such as stretching and flexing in a standing position are fine if you can do them in a relaxed way while breathing naturally.

In addition, hepatitis patients should avoid overexertion. With a tendency toward a low level of blood sugar, hepatitis sufferers are more likely to tire easily. They should, therefore, limit their total amount of therapeutic exercise, excluding *Ch'i Kung* and leisurely walking, to no more than ½ hour. This exercise may be divided into 2 sessions, 1 in the morning and 1 in the afternoon.

It is important to remember that your exercise should proceed slowly and gradually. Do not perform exercise either on an empty stomach or right after a meal.

EDITOR'S NOTE: Any of the following symptoms are also signs that should be read DO NOT EXERCISE: fever of any degree, fatigue, loss of appetite, nausea or pain in the liver area.

Young people who have chronic hepatitis or post-hepatitis syndrome may exercise with a physical education class if they follow the guidelines just given. One group of college students notably improved their health after 6 months of exercises. They had increased appetites, greater physical strength and better mental spirit. Most, if not all, of the students improved their liver functions.

After recovery from hepatitis, you can increase the amount of exercise you do to your pre-disease level once your liver has returned to normal and providing that no other symptoms have shown up.

Generally speaking, a person who has an enlarged liver should avoid strenuous exercises even if the liver is functioning normally. Mild exercises such as easy stretching and calisthenics, badminton and *Tai Chi Chuan* are permitted, but you must keep an eye on your condition. If you don't note any unusual reactions after 1 month's close monitoring, your liver enlargement is probably within normal limits. Check with your doctor. And for the sake of caution, you should continue monitoring your own health. If you find you feel uncomfortable and tired after a small amount of exercise, you should cease exercising temporarily and seek further diagnosis.

Diagnosing and Treating Acute Abdominal Pain

It's often hard to pin down the cause of acute abdominal pain. A common problem, it can be caused by functional disturbances in the organs of the abdomen. It may be caused by defective organs, either inside or outside the abdomen.

Sudden spasmodic pains in the abdomen are frequently triggered by stomach and intestinal cramping. Persistent abdominal pains may be the result of inflammation. Either inflammation or spasm may cause occasional sharp pains. If the pain comes from cramping, it can frequently be relieved by rubbing and pressing the spot that hurts.

When the pains are confined to a certain area, they may indicate an inflammation. If they are accompanied by involuntary muscular tension, it may be inflammation of the peritoneum —the membrane that lines the abdominal cavity and surrounds the abdominal organs. This is a life-threatening condition, and immediate surgery may be necessary.

Fixing the site of the pain can provide valuable diagnostic information. If the pain originates in the middle of the upper abdomen, stomach ailments may be to blame. If it is in the right upper abdomen, liver or gallbladder diseases are suggested. But angina (heart pain) and even heart attacks may cause pain in the upper abdomen. Intermittent pain around the navel, may be caused by ascariasis—an infection of the bowels by roundworms (far more common in undeveloped countries than in the United States).

A frequent cause of pain in the lower right hand corner of the abdomen is appendicitis. Pain originating in the lower left hand corner of the abdomen, may suggest dysentery, especially when accompanied by diarrhea and blood and pus in the stool. When the patient is female, lower abdominal pain may also be caused by gynecological or menstrual problems.

Obviously abdominal pain can be complicated and difficult to interpret. Therefore, a thorough medical evaluation should be performed before you decide whether massage or medicine should be used.

If massage is chosen you may find that massaging an acupuncture point that is far away from the abdomen is the best method. Besides being effective, massaging an acupuncture point does not have the side effects frequently associated with drugs. And it often stops spasmodic stomach and intestinal pain faster than many drugs. After massage, if the pain persists, the patient should immediately consult a physician.

Here are complete directions for two indigestion-relieving massages:

1. Have someone massage the acupuncture points on your Foot-Greater *Yang*-Bladder meridian (located on both sides of the thoracic vertebrae). (See Fig. 72.) A combination of pushing, rubbing, lifting and holding motions should be

used. As you lie stomach down, the masseur presses with the tip and upper portion of the thumb against the selected acupuncture points. Rhythmical rubbing and pushing against the points with the thumb in a circular motion is best. The speed should be 40 to 60 pulses per minute. Pressure should be applied gradually.

If pain persists the lifting and holding method can be used. This method involves lifting and holding the points with all five fingers for 3 to 5 times each. The amount of pressure is about right when you first feel a sore sensation.

2. Or pinch and knead the three acupuncture points called *Tsu San Li*, *Wei Chuan* and *Shun San* (See Fig. 73 and Fig. 74) with a rotating motion. Press each point at brief intervals with the tip of your thumb. The pressure should be increased gradually and never applied abruptly. Continue the massage until the point feels sore and numb.

If greater pressure seems desirable, use a fast-moving, vibrating motion. Pressing and kneading the *Tsu San Li* point as hard and deeply as possible is a very effective pain killer. If *Tsu San Li* is chosen as the site for the massage and if you can get someone else to do the massage, you should lie on your back. On the other hand, when *Wei Chuan* and *Shun San* are used, you should rest on your stomach. You can also massage the three acupuncture points yourself using the techniques described.

Abdominal pain may also be relieved by massaging *Ha Ku*, which is located at the first joint below the tip of the index finger, and the point 3 inches below your navel. Self-massage, however, is not as effective as massage performed by another person.

If you suffer abdominal pain during exercise, you should immediately reduce the level of exercise intensity. Breathe deeply a few times

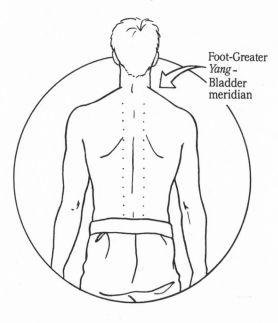

Foot-Greater *Yang* - Bladder meridian

Figure 72. *Acupuncture meridians*

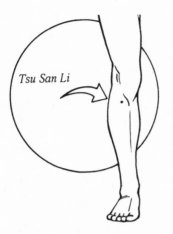

Figure 73. *The* Tsu San Li *point*

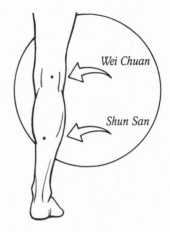

Figure 74. *The* Wei Chuan *and* Shun San *points*

and press and squeeze the painful spot. After this treatment, the pain will usually ease up or even stop. If it does not, you can usually get rid of the pain simply by terminating the exercise. If the problem persists, try the acupressure techniques listed for other abdominal pains. Remember that severe or persistent pain should be evaluated by a physician.

Healing Exercises for Inflammations of the Intestine and Colon

Although chronic enteritis, an inflammation of the intestine, can occur alone, it is frequently accompanied by chronic inflammation of the colon or of the stomach.

The most obvious symptom of enteritis is chronic diarrhea, occurring most often in the early morning or after a meal. The sufferer may feel a mild pain around the navel and become conscious of a fluid movement inside the intestines.

When enteritis is accompanied by colitis, an inflammation of the colon, constipation, diarrhea, pain in the colon, passage of pus, mucus, blood and undigested foods with the stools may occur. The degree of severity of chronic enteritis and chronic colitis may vary considerably. If untreated, the diseases may last from a few years to 30 or more years and cause gradual deterioration of the whole body.

The body's inability to absorb adequate protein, vitamins and other nutrients due to impairment of digestion can affect the nervous system as well as metabolism of foodstuffs. Both, in turn, may aggravate the disease.

Healing exercise can help the body absorb nutrients, can strengthen organs and can help regulate the functioning of the nervous system. These benefits contribute to resistance to disease. To work well, therapeutic exercise should be combined with medicine and performed only before the disease has reached a critical stage.

To recover from chronic enteritis and colitis, you must have faith in the exercise and practice it regularly. In the beginning, you may practice *Fang Sung Kung* (see page 44), in the lying-down position. Practice this exercise 20 to 30 minutes a time, 2 or 3 times a day. After performing this exercise, massage your abdomen with your palms and pinch and rub your stomach area with the thumbs.

When you are in recovery, you may practice *Tai Chi Chuan* in addition to other types of exercise. To get the most therapeutic benefit, you should do these exercises 2 or 3 times a day for at least 20 minutes per session.

Ch'i Kung and Gastroptosis

Unless the symptoms are very obvious, some patients may not even recognize that they have gastroptosis.* When the disease has progressed further and the stomach has fallen from its regular place and descends to the abdominal cavity, the patient may experience headache, dizziness, indigestion, constipation, proneness to fatigue and distension of the abdomen. These symptoms are the result of slow movement through the stomach and intestines, obstruction in the digestive process and an overall weakened physical condition.

There is a close relationship between gastroptosis and the patient's overall physical condition. Gastroptosis sufferers are likely to be slim

---

*Gastroptosis, or fallen stomach, is recognized both by traditional and modern Chinese doctors as a real and serious illness. Western doctors, however, consider the concept that out-of-place organs indicate sickness in the same scientific category as telling the future from a crystal ball. The exercises offered here for gastroptosis, however, are useful for anyone seeking to improve and strengthen health.

and physically weak. The ligaments inside their abdominal cavities are loose—too weak to hold the stomach in place. The slackness of abdominal muscles also causes the stomach to drop. Nutritional deficiencies and consequent weight loss also contribute to gastroptosis. Changes in the shape and dimension of the abdominal cavity after childbirth may also lead to the development of the condition.

The treatment for gastroptosis aims to improve the patient's stamina, strengthen the abdominal muscles and insure an adequate level of nutrition. *Ch'i Kung* and therapeutic gymnastics can also be of great help in relieving gastroptosis.

Ch'i Kung as a therapy for gastroptosis has been well received in China because it both improves the body's condition and increases the patient's appetite. It can also improve the process of digestion and increase the elasticity of the smooth muscles within the stomach and intestines.

Clinical observations in China have shown that after a period of *Ch'i Kung* therapy the stomach moved upward in varying degrees. Symptoms such as indigestion, abdominal pain, bloating and belching also disappeared.

In treating gastroptosis, both *Ch'iang Chuang Kung* (invigorating) and *Nei Yang Kung* (nourishing) techniques may be used. Emphasis should be placed on the lying-on-the-back position. If the condition of gastroptosis is serious, you can support your buttocks with a cushion and bend your legs at the knees. After your condition improves, you may employ the lying-on-the-side position as well as the sitting position. Don't forget to use abdominal breathing. Your breathing should be soft, gentle and relaxed.

In using therapeutic gymnastics to treat gastroptosis, you should emphasize strengthening the abdominal muscles. The gymnastics recommended earlier for treating constipation may also be used for treating gastroptosis.

Obesity

There are two types of obesity: the kind arising from external factors (exogenous) and the kind caused internally (endogenous). Exogenous obesity comes from overeating coupled with a lack of involvement in physical activity. Endogenous obesity is brought about by deficiency in the functioning of the pituitary, thyroid and other glands.

The incidence of endogenous obesity is very low. It accounts for only 3 percent of all cases. Therapeutic exercise can have only a small beneficial effect on this kind of overweight.

On the other hand, healing exercise can be very effective in treating exogenous obesity, which is by far the most common form of obesity. Don't expect your weight to fall from exercise alone, though. You must follow a controlled diet at the same time.

There's evidence that the obese have a tendency to store carbohydrates as fat (rather than convert them into the more readily burned glycogen, a body sugar), more efficiently than the thin. With less glycogen available to be burned, the overweight are more likely to feel hungry and overeat again. In addition, they become less and less likely to exercise because of the breathing and other problems they experience when they try. Therefore, if you notice a steady increase in your weight, you should intervene to bring it under control early.

A careful and conscientious healing exercise program for treating the overweight cannot only reduce fat, but can also help treat problems often found with the condition such as constipation, hemorrhoids, bloating, and weak heart and lungs.

Because of the complex nature of obesity, you should seek the guidance of a doctor when deciding upon an exercise program. The following series of exercises should be considered. They have been recommended by Chinese doctors and may best be practiced in the early morning.

Nei Chuang Kung
(Internal Strength Exercises) Set A

1. Stand with your feet a shoulder width apart, your toes turned very slightly inward and your arms at your sides. With the backs of your hands facing your thighs, lift your arms gracefully with your elbows bent, turning your palms until, when they reach chest level, they face up. As you do this, breathe in deeply. (See Fig. 75.)

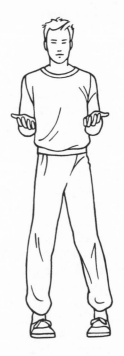

Figure 75. *Standing exercise for internal strength*

Knocking at the Gate of Life

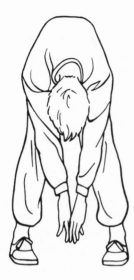

Figure 76. *Bending exercise for internal strength*

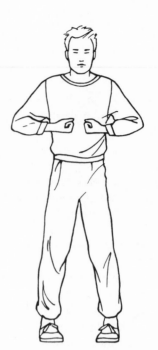

Figure 77. *Raising a heavy weight for internal strength*

2. With the backs of your hands facing each other, bend forward as far as you can without pain, as shown in Fig. 76. As you bend, say "huh!" and exhale completely.

3. Clench each hand into a fist as you stand with your arms at your sides. Raise your hands as if you were lifting a heavy object with the tops of your fists. Turn your fists so that your fingers face up as your hands reach chest level and inhale deeply. (See Fig. 77).

4. Standing with your fists at your sides, fingers facing front, lift your arms straight out to the sides as you exhale. (See Fig. 78a.)

5. While holding your arms out to the side as in step 4, inhale. Then exhale as you rotate the backs of your fists forward with your thumbs toward the floor. (See Fig. 78b.)

6. Still standing with your arms out, inhale again, and then exhale as you turn your fists until your fingers are on top. (See Fig. 78c.)

7. Inhale and bring your arms down from the position in step 6. Press your fists hard against your abdomen to aid your deep exhalation as shown in Fig. 78d.

8. Relax your hands and let your arms hang naturally. Breathe in and out 3 times before repeating the series just described. Depending on your level of fitness, you may repeat this from 10 to 30 times.

Nei Chuang Kung
(Internal Strength Exercises) Set B

1. Position your feet as if you were taking a long step, left foot forward with the knee slightly bent. The distance between the heel of the front

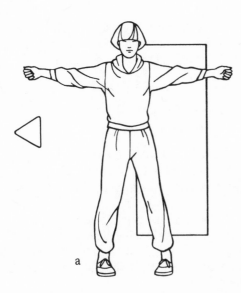

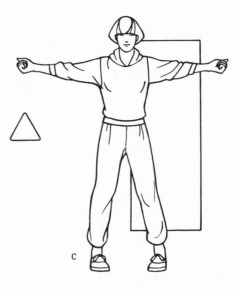

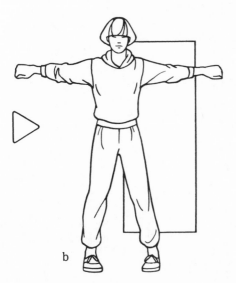

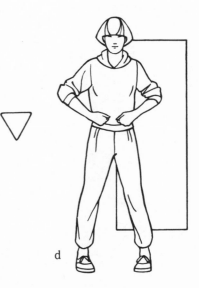

Figure 78. *An internal strengthening sequence*

foot and the toes of the rear foot should be approximately 2 feet. The space defined by your insteps should not exceed 18 inches. The toes of your front foot should face forward but those of the rear foot should turn slightly out. Keep both feet in place during this exercise, with your weight divided between them.

2. With your feet positioned, turn your body slightly to the right and let your eyes follow the movement. Bring your hands up in front of your chest with the backs facing each other and your fingers pointing up as shown in Fig. 79a.

3. Let your arms swoop gracefully downward. Then stretch your left hand out in front of you as you extend your right arm back. (See Fig. 79b.)

4. Turn your body slowly to the left, keeping your eyes level as they follow the turn. You should end up in the exact reverse of the position in step 2. Repeat the same moves as in step 3. The only difference is that your right leg and arm are now in front. Repeat first to the right, then to the left. Work up to 100 alternating repetitions.

Nei Chuang Kung
(Internal Strength Exercises) Set C

1. Stand naturally with your feet parallel to each other about a shoulder width apart. Breathe deeply through your nose for 1 or 2 minutes.

2. Do deep knee bends. As you squat, exhale fully, pressing both hands against your abdomen. Inhale as you rise. Do this 10 to 20 times. Afterward, take a leisurely walk for 10 to 20 minutes.

If they are in good health, obese patients may also jog, swim, take cold water baths, sunbathe and play ball.

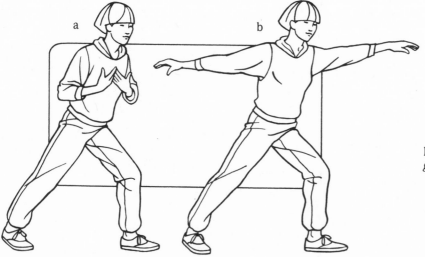

Figure 79. *Gain strength, grace and balance*

Can Fat Be Reduced by Massaging the Abdomen?

For a long time, many people believed that fat in the abdomen could be reduced simply by massaging that region. This is simply not true.

In order to understand why fat cannot be reduced by massage, it is necessary to understand how fat accumulated in the abdomen in the first place. Usually, the total percentage of fat in the body of an average man is approximately 18 percent of his weight. But when a physically inactive person overindulges in eating, the body absorbs more nutrients than it needs. At the same time, the lack of exercise prevents the body from using up the extra unnecessary calories. Excessive sugars and proteins not consumed by the body are transformed into fats. And the abdominal wall tends to become the main depot for excessive fat. The overall result is an overweight problem.

Some studies have shown that when a sedentary person overeats, fat may be absorbed at a rate in excess of ½ ounce of body weight a day. If the trend continues, 1 pound is added each month — 12 pounds per year.

Obviously, the best way to prevent fat accumulating in the body is to make sure there is a proper balance between food intake and physical exercise. Habits of eating excessively and doing little or no exercise should be avoided.

If excessive fat has already been accumulated in the abdomen or other parts of the body, the most sensible way to reduce it is to exercise. The stored fat can be consumed as energy.

Two conditions must be met to lose weight through exercise. Not only must you become more active, but you need to reduce food intake, too. For exercise, walking, jogging, playing ball, swimming or hiking are all good. Naturally, these exercises should not be performed if you have other complications. Obese individuals with coronary heart disease or hypertension should refrain from exercises of high intensity. They should make dietary control the primary focus of their weight reduction program and participate in a moderate exercise program under the guidance of a physician.

CHAPTER SIX

Healing the Nervous System

康

Illnesses that affect the nervous system produce a broader range of symptoms and problems than afflictions in any other system in the body. From the moping disinterest in life, poor appetite and insomnia that characterize the depressed to an actual inability to walk, nervous system disorders have serious and unpleasant impacts on our lives. But whether they are ordinary problems such as occasional insomnia or motion sickness or the serious damages resulting from polio and spinal injury, this chapter presents exercises that may be able to help.

Depression

Should depression be treated with rest or exercise? If the depression is caused by exhaustion, rest and sleep are key to revitalizing nerve cells in the thinking parts of the brain. But Chinese doctors have noted again and again that rest alone is not enough. It's also important that the depressed person improve physical fitness, which will enhance the ability to cope with both home and work situations.

Exercise also helps cure depression. It's not just a way to strengthen the patient for life after recovery. During workouts, muscles and joints feed a steady stream of neural impulses to the central nervous system. These transmissions have a regulating effect on the nervous system, medical professionals believe. Muscle training is, in essence, nervous system training, these doctors say. Physical exercise actually conditions the nervous system.

In addition, physical activity helps divert the depressive's attention away from obsessive involvement with problems. This helps improve the emotional state, and therefore, also lessens other symptoms.

Rest, exercise and recreation—all must be emphasized in the treatment of the depressive.

How effectively exercise will heal will vary from person to person because each individual's problem is different. Those who suffer from chronic tiredness due to mental strain, overwork and physical inactivity will benefit the most from healing exercise. People who are in a physically weakened condition as well as mentally exhausted should get plenty of rest. The exercise for them is *Ch'i Kung*, specifically the relaxation breathing technique *Fang Sung Kung*. (See page 44.) Do not, however, practice *Ch'i Kung* for overly long sessions.

If depression is an outgrowth of other diseases, then treatment should begin with those diseases before an attempt is made to relieve the depression.

Exercise Systems for Depression

The best healing exercises for treating depression are *Tai Chi Chuan, Ch'i Kung*, massage, leisurely walking, hikes and expeditions and cold water bathing. Of these, *Tai Chi Chuan* appears to be the most effective.

Tai Chi Chuan: In recent years the Chinese have used *Tai Chi* widely and successfully in treating depression. This exercise offers special benefits because it calls for mental and emotional tranquility. It requires full concentration so that what the mind imagines, the body becomes. Because of its mental and spiritual demands, *Tai Chi* conditions the nervous system and helps feelings of calm and peace grow. After a reasonable period of practice, *Tai Chi* will often cure the problems of mental distraction and irritability.

Tai Chi Chuan is rather complicated to learn and it takes times to become proficient, but it is worth it. The best way to learn is to take the technique step by step—from the simplest to the most complex and from the easiest to the most difficult. And as you study and practice, keep in mind these three key words that describe the movements of *Tai Chi—calm, loose, slow*

Ch'i Kung: In traditional Chinese medicine, *Ch'i Kung* is noted for its effectiveness in treating diseases characterized by the qualities known as emptiness, weariness, deficiency and injury. *Ch'i Kung* nourishes *yuen ch'i*—vital energy—and builds up inner strength. It is a good medicine for depression. And many clinics in China have reported success with its use.

Ch'i Kung works on depression mainly because it produces mental quietness. In this state, the exerciser "turns off" cortical activity—active thinking, worrying and fretting—and weary nerve cells gain a chance to revitalize.

It is recommended that the *Ch'iang Chuang Kung* technique (see page 46) in the sitting position be employed by the depressed individual. The physically weak may adopt the lying-down position and the physically fit may perform the exercise while standing. Whatever position is chosen, the goal of the exercise remains a state of mental quietness. You may practice *Ch'i Kung* for 30-minute sessions, 2 to 3 times a day.

Massage: Massage can be very effective when performed by patients themselves. Often depression is accompanied by other symptoms. For headache, rub your face with the same kind of brisk motion you use when brushing your teeth. Also massage the acupuncture points around your eyes. (See page 65.) For dizziness, gently thump your head all over, snapping both your index and middle fingers against it while you cover your ears with your palms. Rubbing the acupuncture point *Yung Ch'uan* (Bubbling Spring) is a very effective remedy for insomnia and anxiety-related palpitations. It is found in the middle of the soles of both your feet.

Leisurely walking, hikes and vacations: A leisurely walk for a distance of 1½ to 2 miles can help regulate the excitation and inhibition processes of the cerebral cortex, reducing symptoms such as headaches and throbbing pains in the temples. And many patients have noticed that their moods and spirits improved as a result of engaging in exercise regularly. For the physically fit person, field trips and excursions also help divert attention away from problems.

Water bathing: A cold water bath is good for the depressed person because of its soothing effects on the nervous system. The best time to take a cold water bath is in the early morning. To begin the process, you may rub your body with warm water. After a few days, you may switch to cool water if you can adapt to it without discomfort. Finally, take a cold water bath or shower

for 30 seconds or 1 minute. Remember, too, that in the summer, swimming is a good exercise for the depressed.

Other exercises: Exercises such as table tennis, basketball, canoeing and similar outdoor exercises are good for the depressed. But for this healing exercise treatment program to be successful, depressed people should remember that physical activity is only one component in the comprehensive treatment program. To be successful, the depressive must at the same time resolve the personal problems that contribute to the neurosis. The depressive should also work on maintaining a proper balance between work and relaxation and developing a spirit of optimism.

The amount of exercise you should do depends on your physical condition. If you're weak, do only *Ch'i Kung* and massage. If you're fit, you may exercise for ½ to 1 hour (not counting the time for *Ch'i Kung*). The physically strong may exercise 1 to 2 hours in both the morning and afternoon. But if you ever experience excessive perspiration, overexcitement or insomnia, you should reduce the amount of exercise.

Have confidence in healing exercise. It and your fighting spirit can combat depression.

Curing Insomnia

Insomnia can be caused by any number of factors. The most common ones, however, are depression and temporary emotional disturbances. For these types of insomnia, sleeping pills are only a temporary cure. To treat the underlying causes, the patient must calm down and inhibit the overstimulated cerebral cortex. An effective way to accomplish this is through healing exercise.

The following exercises can be performed individually or consecutively:

1. Before bedtime, take a leisurely walk for 5 or 10 minutes or perform one set of *Tai Chi Chuan*. After you have calmed down, go to bed.

2. Before bedtime, perform self-massage either sitting or lying on your back. Cover your body with a blanket if the room temperature is low. Massage the body all over as if you were taking a dry bath. First rub your face gently with both hands. Then, massage your left arm with your right hand and vice versa. Next, rub the chest and abdominal regions. Your hand movement should be slow and light. Finally, massage the acupuncture point *Yung Ch'uan*, which is located in the middle of the sole of the foot. Continue massaging until you feel calm and peaceful. Usually 10 minutes of self-massage will do it. You'll feel tired and sleepy. So relax your body and go to bed. The type of massage you just gave yourself is valuable because it frequently produces a calming and hypnotic effect.

3. Perform *Ch'i Kung* just before bedtime. You may perform either *Fang Sung Kung* or *Ch'iang Chuang Kung* (see pages 44 and 46). Or you can simply lie on the right side of your body and let your muscles get loose. Then let your mind follow the rhythm of your breathing until you fall into slumber. Since the purpose of this exercise is to induce sleep, the amount of time spent is not important. Generally, it takes about 10 minutes or so before you feel sleepy.

You may combine this exercise with other techniques such as soaking your feet in warm water for 20 or 30 minutes just before bedtime. And be sure not to engage in mental work for 30 minutes before going to sleep. If you awaken after falling asleep, just perform the same exercise again until you fall asleep once more.

Preventing Motion Sickness

Some individuals feel dizzy and nauseated whenever they ride in a car or a boat. They may even perspire, grow pale or vomit. These people are susceptible to carsickness and seasickness. Flying in an airplane may also cause some individuals to display symptoms. Medically, these conditions are called motion sickness—any illness caused by irregular, repeated movement of the body. Some estimates say that more than 80 percent of first-time boat passengers suffer from seasickness.

The explanation lies deep within the ear. The human ear consists of the external ear shell, the middle ear and the internal ear. The internal ear is located in the temporal bone. Within the internal ear lies the vestibule, containing the receptors for position and movement.

When a person rides in an airplane or car, these receptors may be jolted by the movement of the vehicle. The vestibular structure must adapt. A person whose vestibule adapts well will not develop carsickness or seasickness. But a person who has a sensitive vestibule is likely to feel seasick or carsick.

Other factors such as overeating, fatigue, fever, insufficient sleep, emotional overstimulation and air pollution can contribute to motion sickness. The odor of gasoline and burning fuel may aggravate the problem.

One easy answer to carsickness or seasickness is to take Dramamine, meclizine or ginger root. But it is also possible to prevent the illness in the first place and avoid drugs. You can practice being a passenger until your vestibule has adapted to the irregular motion. Many sailors and drivers have overcome their motion sickness simply by exposing themselves to the situation. However, if this is not practical, there are other ways to avoid carsickness or seasickness.

The best approach to preventing motion sickness is to engage in exercises that involve body balance—such as roller skating, rope swinging, rope ladder climbing, the uneven parallel bars and simply rolling around on an exercise mat. These exercises can improve the adaptability of the vestibule to irregular motion.

The following two exercises from the *Pa Kua Ch'ang* (The Palm of the Eight Diagrams), which require no equipment, have also proved exceptionally useful in preventing motion sickness.

Palms-up posture: Holding your hands with palms near your shoulders and bending your knees slightly, you will walk patterns on the floor. First walk in a big circle, spiraling inward until you are simply circling one point on the floor. Then walk around an imaginary square, 4 feet on a side, several times. Then follow the sides of a 3-foot triangle. Finally, turn yourself in a circle until you become slightly dizzy, keeping your palms up and knees bent. When you recover, turn in the other direction.

Circling with the upper body: Stand with your feet slightly more than a shoulder width apart. Hold the back of the head with both hands with your fingers laced. Then moving clockwise from the waist make a large circle in front of your body until you feel a little bit dizzy. Repeat the motion counterclockwise. (See Fig. 80.)

Treating Sciatica with Exercise

There are many possible causes of sciatica. This troublesome nerve condition usually causes a sharp pain in the buttocks, which radiates into one leg and often into the foot. It is frequently associated with weakness and numbness. A herniated (slipped) disk, osteoarthritis of the spine and sciatic neuritis (inflammation of the sciatic nerve) can all cause this problem.

The last-mentioned form of sciatica can come from the common cold, the absorption of toxins from the environment or inflammation of tissues in surrounding areas, say Chinese doctors. Fortunately, this type of sciatica does respond well to healing exercise. But you should not exercise during acute attacks of sciatic neuritis. However, massage and gymnastic exercises can definitely help during the chronic stage.

For the kind of massage that is most helpful in cases of chronic sciatic neuritis, you will need to prepare a simple but special tool. Wrap or roll a wooden rod in a number of layers of cloth to

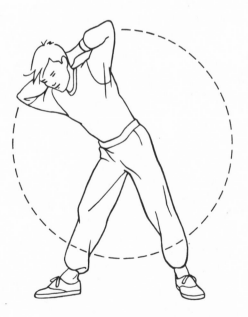

Figure 80. *Circling with the upper body*

cushion it. Then tap yourself, starting at the waist and moving around to your back. Do your hips and legs. Each muscle group should receive 5 or 10 minutes' attention. Repeat this tapping 3 to 5 times a day.

After performing massage, the patient in the early stages of recovery may do the following exercises while lying in bed:

1. While resting on your back with your legs bent, press your knees together. Then try to separate them with your hands while using the opposing muscle group to continue to hold them against each other. Continue for 30 seconds.

2. As you lie on your back with your legs bent, straighten each leg in turn, keeping your thighs parallel, and hold your leg aloft 30 seconds. Reverse legs.

3. As you lie on your side with a slight bend at the hip and your painful side up, move your affected leg backward and forward gently for 1 minute or so.

4. As you sit on the bed, leaning back on your hands for support, extend and bend each leg in turn. Repeat 8 times, or fewer if you become uncomfortable. (See Fig. 81.)

After you have improved your condition and feel somewhat better, you can continue with the following exercises:

5. While sitting in a chair with your legs slightly bent, place your hands on your legs. Bend forward from the waist and let your hands slide down over your legs to your feet as shown in Fig. 82. Repeat 4 times.

6. While sitting on a bed with your legs stretched out in front of you, lean forward gently and try to touch your toes. Repeat several times.

7. While standing and holding onto something sturdy, swing your affected leg forward and backward easily. Keep your knee fairly straight. Continue for up to 5 minutes.

8. With your hands on your hips, put your weight on your right foot, bend your right leg

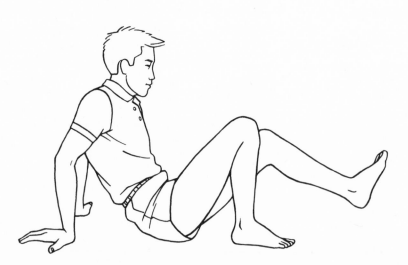

Figure 81. *Sitting exercise for healing sciatica*

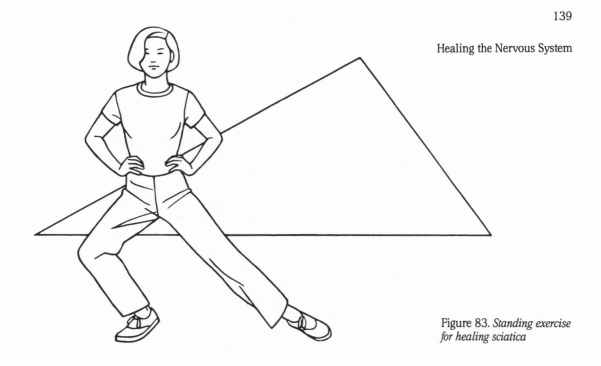

Figure 83. *Standing exercise for healing sciatica*

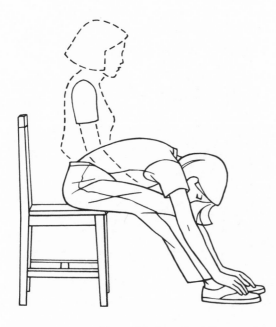

Figure 82. *An anti-sciatica exercise*

and extend your left foot to the left side as shown in Fig. 83. Stand up again and repeat with the other leg. Do 8 bends on each side.

9. While standing with your hands on your hips, lean slightly forward from the waist and then backward. Repeat 8 times. Gradually increase the distance you bend.

If your sciatica is caused by a slipped disk, there are different exercises that should help you. Remember to base the amount of exercise you do on your level of fitness and wellness.

If your problem is mild, your slipped disk may return to its original position after some days of bed rest. To speed up the healing, you should receive massage from a physical therapist. And do this exercise: while standing up straight with your feet together, hold onto a horizontal bar over your head. Gently twist your body from side to side—the movement will be mostly in your arms and sholders. Your torso remains straight as it turns from left to right. Repeat this exercise 2 or 3 times a day.

If after 10 days your condition has not appreciably improved, discontinue the exercise program and seek other forms of treatment.

Brain Concussion

Head injury can sometimes lead to brain concussion—a sort of shock to the brain. After rest and therapy, some patients completely recover from the trauma. Others may still suffer aftereffects such as dizziness, headache, fatigue, depression, inability to concentrate and lack of strength in the limbs.

Healing exercises can be of definite help in relieving these symptoms, particularly when used in conjunction with any needed medicine. The exercises designed for people with depression can also be practiced by patients suffering from the aftermath of brain concussion, but you should cut down on the number of repetitions. *Ch'i Kung* can also help. Emphasize relaxation breathing techniques (see page 44). Leisurely walking in the fresh air and gymnastic exercises, especially set two of *Pa Tuan Chin* (see page 26), are good.

Table tennis is recommended for patients who are physically healthy. Listening to music while doing exercise tends to relax the nervous system. And self-massage of the head, either by rubbing or gentle tapping, can also lessen some symptoms.

Help for Paralytics

In the past, some scholars outside China believed that very little could be done to help people who'd suffered paralysis on one side of their bodies regain the ability to move the affected muscles. This is simply not true. Healing exercise, physical therapy and other forms of rehabilitation can make a difference in the speed and degree of recovery if they are used at the appropriate time.

The author of this book has observed that in two groups of hemiplegics (paralyzed on one side of the body) whose conditions were caused by cerebral hemorrhage, 90 percent of those who did healing exercise learned to walk again either alone or with support. Only 62 percent of those who did not participate in exercise regained this crucial skill.

Hemiplegia is most frequently caused by injury to the motor center of the brain. A hemorrhage, thrombosis or embolism is usually the villain. Healing exercise begun while the patient

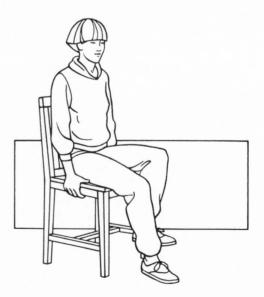

Figure 84. *Seated marching*

is in the process of recovery and practiced persistently can make a marked difference in the speed and degree of improvement.

Healing exercises for hemiplegics can be divided into three stages: in stage one, the patient works on regaining the ability to sit down and stand up. Massage from a medical professional is helpful and so is manipulation of the affected limbs by a physical therapist. But in addition, the patient should begin working to gain mastery of the following progressive set of exercises.

EDITOR'S NOTE: The amount of exercise for recovering paralysis patients should be kept light. Be careful not to overburden the cardiovascular system. And exercise safely. Have someone around when you are practicing standing and walking drills.

1. While lying down, bend and stretch both ankles and toes. Then bend and stretch your leg, first at the hip, then at the knee.

2. At first with the help of another person and then later by yourself, get from the bed into a chair next to the bed.

3. While sitting in a chair, lift each foot in turn and pretend to walk as shown in Fig. 84.

4. Raise yourself from a sitting position in a chair by holding onto the back of another chair placed in front of you as shown in Fig. 85.

5. Stand upright for a minute or two holding onto a chair or the bedpost for support.

6. Stand up alone near a support but without holding on for several minutes.

7. Stand up completely without support.

In stage two the patient regains the ability to walk and increases the mobility of the upper body, particularly the fingers.

The basic steps for training to walk are as follows:

1. While holding onto a support, shift your weight from left to right. (See Fig. 86.)

2. Holding onto a support, walk steadily in place. (See Fig. 87.)

3. Walk sideways with support. (See Fig. 88.)

4. Walk with the support of a wheeled walker.

5. Walk with a cane.

6. Walk alone.

The basic techniques for regaining the use of the hands are as follows:

1. Use massage to reduce finger stiffness. Manipulate the fingers, using physical therapy techniques.

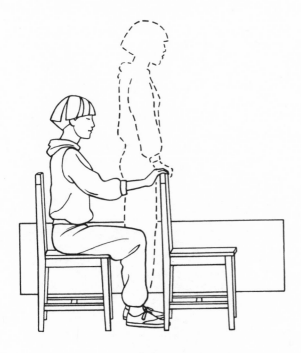

Figure 85. *Practicing standing*

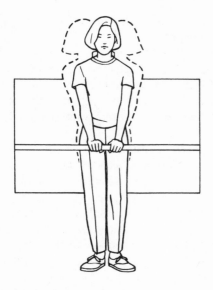

Figure 86. *Shifting weight*

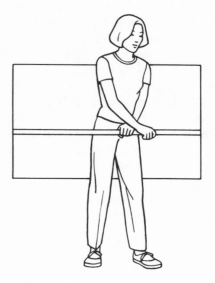

Figure 88. *Walking sideways*

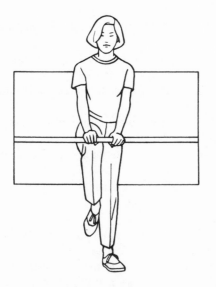

Figure 87. *Walking in place*

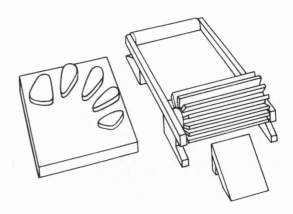

Figure 89. *Finger-strengthening devices*

2. Train your paralyzed fingers to bend, stretch, close and open with small mechanical aids such as the finger-dividing board and the finger roller. (See Fig. 89.) The small piece to the right is for supporting the heel of your hand as you roll your fingers.

3. Develop fine motor skills by engaging in knot tying, button fastening, writing and moving counters on an abacus.

The purpose of stage three is to restore the basic skills used in daily life.

You can speed up recovery of your proficiency at walking by practicing lifting your feet high off the ground while walking, walking in long steps, walking over obstructions, taking lengthy walks, walking on slopes and climbing stairs.

If you are progressing well in recovering the use of your arm and your hand, you may try exercises that require more skill and adroitness such as dribbling a basketball and shooting baskets. Exercises that improve the mobility of the hands such as knitting are also excellent.

Healing Exercises for Paraplegics

Paraplegia is paralysis of the lower half of the body. It is usually caused by injury to the spinal cord.

In China, healing exercise plays an important role in the treatment of paraplegia. The following are some techniques to help train the paraplegic to stand up during the recovery period. These techniques are designed primarily for patients who are recovering from their injury. Patients whose spinal cords have been severely damaged and who need surgery should not do exercises until after they have had their operations.

Here are the progressive exercises to help paraplegics to regain the ability to stand. The first step is to partially rise up from your bed, almost to a sitting position, but leaning back on your arms. After you have become accustomed to this position, sit up on the bed, leaning against the headboard with your legs stretched out straight. Then sit alone on the bed without support. Finally, sit on the edge of the bed.

During the early stage of this sitting training, you may sometimes feel dizzy due to inadequate blood circulation in the head. Two strategies may be used to correct this problem. One thing that may help is to move around in bed and change resting positions frequently when not training. The other alternative is mechanical: it may actually help if you wear a snug belt when practicing. This may prevent a sudden rush of blood from the upper body and brain to the legs and abdominal cavity.

Once you have learned to sit on the edge of the bed, you can begin training in getting up. But first you must strengthen lumbar and shoulder regions. The following exercises are designed for that purpose:

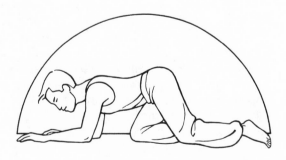

Figure 90. *Recovering from paralysis*

1. Raise your body from a lying-on-your-stomach-in-bed position and crawl forward as shown in Fig. 90. If it is not possible to get up on your knees, simply raise the upper portion of your body and drag yourself forward.

2. In a crawling position as in step 1, attempt to shift your hip joints to move your legs slightly forward and backward. You may use short staffs under your arms for support.

Once you have built up some strength, you may stand up by sliding off the bed. (See Fig. 91.) The next step is to lean against a reclining board. (See Fig. 92.) Once you feel secure with that, you can stand up near a wall with the support of crutches and a physical therapist to hold your knees. (See Fig. 93.) After that, stand up near a wall with crutches by yourself. (See Fig. 94.) You can then proceed to standing up at the parallel bars. (See Fig. 95.) Do more practice standing alone with crutches. Then stand holding onto someone for support. Finally, you will be able to stand up alone.

When you can stand up with support, begin following these sequential steps. First, try walking between the parallel bars or using an adjustable walker. (See Fig. 96.) Then walk with crutches with a therapist to help you control your knees. (See Fig. 97.) Then walk unassisted with crutches. From that point, progress to walking with two canes—then with one cane. At last, walk alone. The third stage of therapeutic exercises designed for hemiplegics (page 141) can also be performed by paraplegics. But remember in all exercises, it is important to protect your knees and have support near the waist so that you don't fall. You can arrange to have someone guard your knees from in front. In China leash-type devices are sometimes fastened to the patient's knees so that a physical therapist can help the patient walk from behind by alternately pulling each leash.

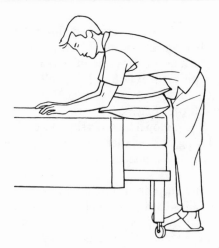

Figure 91. *Sliding off bed*

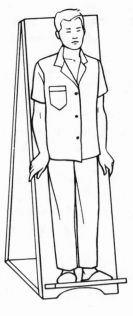

Figure 92. *Using reclining board*

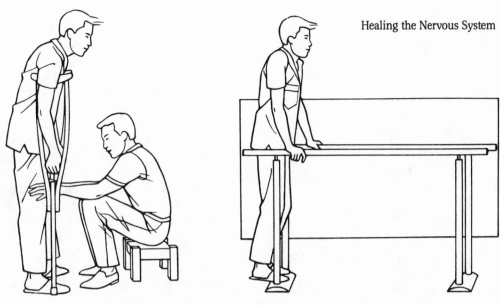

Figure 93. *First time with crutches*

Figure 95. *Standing at parallel bars*

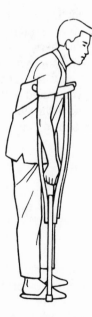

Figure 94. *Standing alone with crutches*

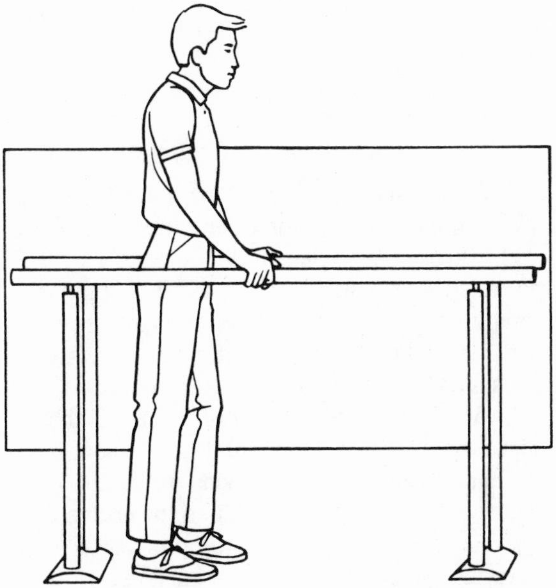

Figure 96. *Walking between parallel bars*

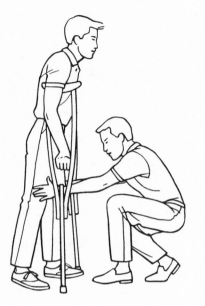

Figure 97. *Starting to walk with crutches*

Some patients will never pass the stage of walking with crutches or other support equipment. To train these patients to use crutches, the so-called four-point walk sequence should be taught. It goes, left foot forward, right crutch forward, right foot forward, left crutch forward. This method is slow but steady.

An alternative is to move both crutches forward at the same time, and then follow by swinging both feet and the body forward. The feet should always remain behind the crutches.

As long as they are in the process of recovering, patients whose paraplegia is caused by inflammation of the spinal cord may also perform the preceding exercises.

Physical Fitness for Paraplegics

Can a patient suffering from incurable paraplegia participate in physical exercise and sports competition? The answer is yes. It isn't even unusual these days for paraplegics to participate in table tennis tournaments and other sports activities in China and elsewhere.

The fact is that the paraplegics can and should do physical exercise. Having lost the use of their legs, it is even more important for them to keep their upper bodies in shape. The proper kinds of exercise can help strengthen muscle groups in the arms, abdomen and lumbar regions. Building strength in this way also builds a sense of self-reliance.

What types of exercise can be performed by patients in wheelchairs? The most suitable are table tennis, shooting baskets, archery, ball throwing and dumbbell exercises. These exercises, particularly archery, not only increase muscle strength in the upper body but can also correct a lateral spinal curvature. If the curvature is to the right, you would pull the bow with your right arm. Done in the clinic, hospital or at home, these exercises also improve balance and coordination.

Epileptic Children and Exercise

During a seizure, some young patients suffer severe convulsions and loss of consciousness. Some adults are reluctant to allow epileptic children to exercise because they fear it may trigger an attack.

Actually, it is desirable for epileptic children to do exercises as long as the exercises are appropriate and safe. These children need both clean air and sunlight. Exercises that are relaxing, slow-paced and simple—such as leisurely walks, field trips, stretching routines, badminton and table tennis—are good for epileptic children.

In order to prevent seizures, exercises that tend to overstimulate the nervous system and exercises that may lead to injury, such as soccer, basketball and sprinting should be avoided. Time-consuming, fatigue-inducing and strenuous exercises are also unsuitable for epileptic children. Any exercises that pose a serious risk of head injury should be bypassed. Epileptic children should not engage in swimming, diving, motorcycling, bicycling, horseriding or mechanical gymnastics. This is the opinion of Chinese physicians.

Paralysis and Therapeutic Exercise

During the Cultural Revolution, medical professionals in China applied the so-called new therapeutic techniques for treating paralysis caused by polio. As a result of their efforts, many children regained their mobility. These techniques are embodied in many healing exercises.

Due to vaccines, polio is rare but not nonexistent in the modern world. A childhood paralysis caused by a degeneration of the motor nerve cells that results in loss of motor function, polio is a dreaded but fortunately now infrequent disease.

But muscles injured by infantile paralysis can be helped to heal with exercise and massage. We will focus on the muscle groups most frequently affected by polio. These are the quad-

riceps muscle of the thigh, the tibial muscles in the calf, the peroneal or fibular muscles in the outer calf, the iliopsoas muscle of the thigh and the muscles of the hip—the gluteus maximus, gluteus medius and gluteus minimus.

To help revitalize these paralyzed muscles, it is important to focus your exercises and massages on the ones that have been most affected.

The quadriceps muscle of the thigh extends the leg. A patient with paralysis here lacks the strength to straighten the knee and extend the lower leg. This patient cannot stand up and walk without support.

Stronger thighs: The quadriceps muscles can be strengthened with these exercises:

1. Sitting down on a flat surface with your legs stretched out straight in front of you, contract the quadriceps muscles to pull your kneecaps

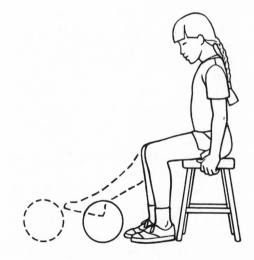

Figure 98. *Kicking ball to recover strength in leg muscles*

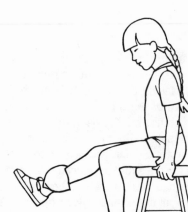

Figure 99. *Lifting small beanbag*

Foot control: Exercises that train the peroneal or fibular muscles develop the ability to turn the foot outward. Some good ones follow:

1. While sitting, try to roll your feet so that the outer edges are lifted off the ground without raising the inner edges.

2. This is a sitting isometric exercise—an exercise that works opposing muscle groups against each other. Here you are to press your knees, ankles and feet together while simultaneously trying to separate them with your hands.

upward. Then relax and let the kneecaps return to their original position. Repeat several times.

2. Sitting in a chair with the affected leg bent, try hard to raise your foot off the ground. Use your hand to help lift it.

3. Sitting in a chair, try as hard as possible to extend your leg without help. Place a ball in front of the leg and try to kick it. (See Fig. 98.)

4. Sitting in a chair, raise your foot with a small weight such as a beanbag draped over it as shown in Fig. 99.

Drawing the foot up: Here are exercises to strengthen the anterior tibial muscles which flex the feet upward:

1. While sitting, hook your foot upward with the help of your hands.

2. While sitting, try hard to hook your foot upward without help.

3. Stand up with support from parallel bars or some other sturdy object. Lift the front part of first one foot and then the other without raising the heel off the ground.

4. Walk on your heels.

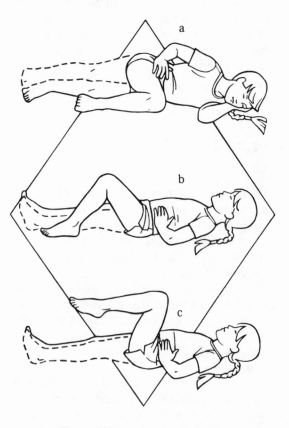

Figure 100. *Leg exercises for healing muscles*

Other thigh and hip helpers: The following exercises strengthen the iliopsoas muscle, which makes it possible to flex the hip and lift the leg:

1. While lying on your side, attempt to swing your thigh forward. (See Fig. 100a.)

2. While lying on your back, bend your leg at the knee and draw your leg up without lifting the heel from the bed. (See Fig. 100b.)

3. While lying on your back, try to bring your bent leg up and flex it over your abdomen. (See Fig. 100c.)

4. While lying on your back, try to lift your leg without bending the knee. (See Fig. 101.)

Hip muscles: The hip muscles move the legs backward and support the pelvis when you're standing. If the hip muscles lack sufficient strength, you won't be able to walk steadily. These exercises are useful for strengthening the muscles of the hip:

1. While lying on your back, contract the muscles of the hip and bring the buttocks together. Your hips will rise slightly.

2. While lying on your stomach, extend and lift your leg backward, without bending your knee. (See Fig. 102.)

3. While lying on your back, move your leg to the side. (See Fig. 103.)

In addition to working on individual muscle groups, the patient should do exercises designed to strengthen the whole body. Exercises to strengthen the arms, shoulders and back shouldn't be neglected. A good overall exercise is simply crawling on the floor.

Other exercises, too, can help train the paralyzed child to stand up. To begin, the child should sit in a kneeling position with buttocks resting on heels. Then the child may gradually switch to standing on his or her knees. He or she can also practice squatting exercises while holding onto the bedstead as shown in Fig. 104.

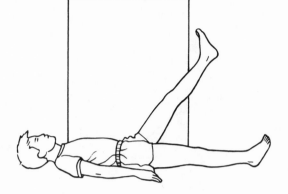

Figure 101. *Leg lift*

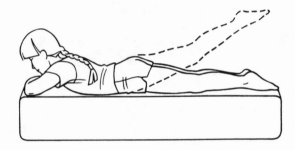

Figure 102. *Strengthening the back and legs*

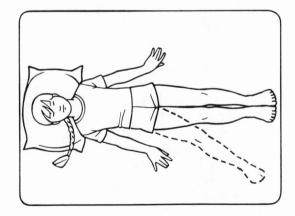

Figure 103. *Building strength in the hip*

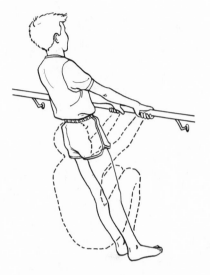

Figure 104. *How to do a squatting exercise*

Exercises that are like play, such as riding a tricycle, should also be encouraged.

When the child is strong enough to begin walking, help by supporting him or her under the arms and walking with him or her. The child can also walk with a cane or a walker. The next step is to walk unassisted on level ground. Practice walking over an obstacle (as in Fig. 105) can also help. Walking in a circle or up and down stairs (as in Fig. 106) can build strength, balance and coordination.

Do walking practice after the exercises for individual muscle groups. Walking periods of 5 to 10 minutes should be broken frequently with rests. Very gradually increase walking time to 20 to 30 minutes a session.

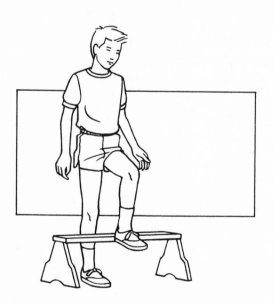

Figure 105. *Stepping over an obstacle*

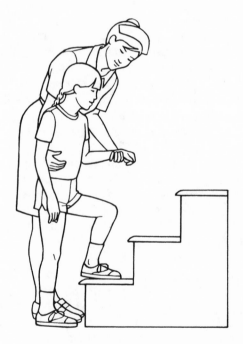

Figure 106. *Relearning the stairs*

CHAPTER SEVEN

Relaxing and Toning Muscles and Bones

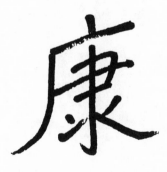

Making you stronger and more flexible is one gift that healing exercise regularly gives. As helpful as it is for diseases of the organs and internal systems, its most immediate impact is on the parts of the body involved in movement—the bones, muscles, ligaments and related tissues. The Chinese have devoted centuries of study to developing the exercises to make these structures strong and to heal them when they are injured.

These healing exercises can help you reverse age. Just as nothing makes you feel older than sore, weak, creaking and painful joints and muscles, nothing contributes to a youthful feeling more than a flexible, strong and eager body. Healing exercise can give you that.

Even if your body has been bent and misshapen by years of misuse, lack of use or disease, healing exercise may be able to help. This chapter tells you how.

Preventing and Easing Arthritis

The movements of *Tai Chi Chuan* involve every important joint in the body. Regular practice of *Tai Chi* keeps both bones and joints healthy. This classic Chinese exercise routine is, therefore, one of the best ways to prevent arthritis. *Tai Chi Chuan* is thoroughly discussed in Chapter Two of this book.

Many people who have already developed arthritis may still be helped by practicing *Tai Chi*. The exercise's effectiveness will depend on how far the disease has advanced and what joints are affected. You should do *Tai Chi* only if you can do it without undue pain.

When arthritis is mild most people will not have extreme pain or stiffness and will be able to use *Tai Chi* as a form of therapy. *Tai Chi* practice at this stage will help improve your overall health as well as the mobility of your joints. But inflammation in the knees, the small of the back, the sacroiliac or other joints that are actively involved in the exercise may serve only to intensify the pain. Patients who have pain in these joints may wish to try out the exercise for a period of time under close medical supervision. If they adapt well and suffer no negative effects, they may continue and expect good results.

Some arthritics do experience pain at the outset, but they later find their pain soothed and their overall health improved. However, if your condition seems to be worsening as a result of the exercise, don't ignore it. Stop exercising—at least temporarily. If you have a significant problem, you may want to consult your doctor about the advantages of exercise for your condition.

How Exercise Can Help Rheumatoid Arthritis

In rheumatoid arthritis the joints are often swollen, painful and stiff. But healing exercise can help improve joint mobility when the condition is

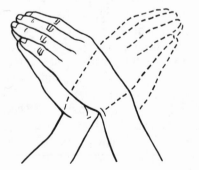

Figure 107. *Flexing the wrists*

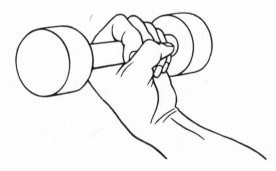

Figure 108. *A dumbbell builds wrists*

chronic. And it can help stop it from becoming acute. Even when there is acute inflammation, exercise can be of benefit. It can also prevent such flareups.

The affected joints need exercise several times a day. Exercise rods—an old broomstick will do—can be especially useful in improving flexibility of the joints. (Some excellent exercises will be described, many requiring no equipment at all.)

Massage and passive exercise of the affected joints can help when other kinds of exercise don't. With smaller joints, such as the finger, wrist, elbow and ankle, start by soaking them in warm water—just about body temperature, 98.6°F. A warm water soak lessens muscle pain and spasm, and it makes your joints easier to move.

After your warm soak of 10 minutes or so, you may try any of the following exercises that apply to your problem joints. If you have a problem with your fingers, clutch a pencil or stick tightly. Then straighten your fingers and palm by flattening your hand against a table or desk.

To improve the flexibility of your wrists, press your palms together in front of your chest. Use each hand in turn to press the other back. (See Fig. 107.) Do this rapidly, and don't be afraid to press fairly hard. A light dumbbell can also be used to build strength and increase mobility in your wrists, as shown in Fig. 108.

To help stiff elbows, try making fists and touching your knuckles to your shoulders. Then fling your arms downward, fingers spread, to about 6 inches outside your thighs. (See Fig. 109a.)

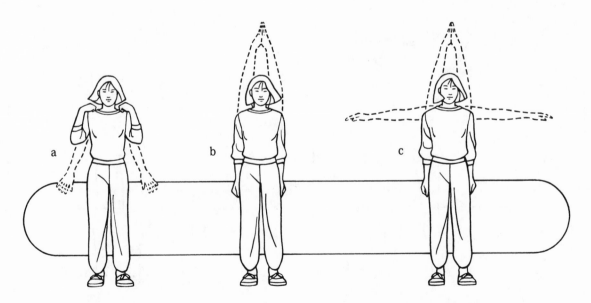

Figure 109. *Strengthening the arms and shoulders*

A good shoulder-loosening exercise is to stand with your arms at your sides, stretch your hands out to the sides and touch your palms together over your head. (See Fig. 109b.)

A variation on this exercise that will also help stiff sore shoulders is to first raise your arms out to the sides only to shoulder level, lower them again and then touch your palms over your head. (See Fig. 109c.)

To increase your shoulders' forward and backward mobility, lace your fingers behind your head as you stand upright, then draw your elbows back to open the shoulders as fully as possible. (See Fig. 110.)

Next, with your fingers laced and the front of your hands against the back of your waist, curl your shoulders forward as if you were trying to make them meet in front of your body. (See Fig. 111.)

For problem ankles, the best exercise is simply to flex, extend and rotate your feet, first in one direction then in another while sitting.

To build hip and knee flexibility, take a long step forward and bend your front leg. With your hands on your hips, draw your elbows back, and thrust your chest forward. Hold this position until your muscles tire. (See Fig. 112.) Alternate legs.

You can also do deep knee bends while holding on to the back of a chair for support. Keep your heels on the floor.

Finally, while holding on to the back of a chair or some other sturdy object, swing your leg back and forth forcefully, as in Fig. 113. Now switch legs.

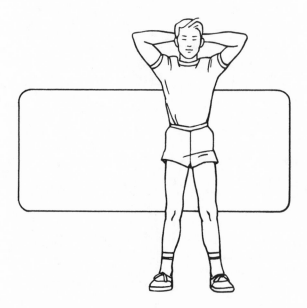

Figure 110. *Opening the shoulder joints*

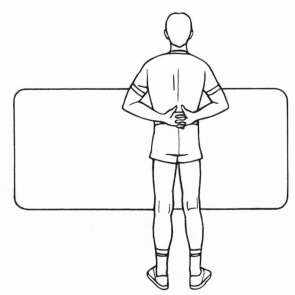

Figure 111. *Curling the shoulders forward*

Each of these exercises may be done 10 to 20 times, preferably at least 2 times a day. In addition, you can massage the affected joints and the surrounding muscles to lessen pain and swelling. Rub and knead the joints lightly, but massage your muscles deeply. About the right amount of time to spend on a massage is 10 to 20 minutes.

Exercises for Spinal Deterioration

When rheumatoid arthritis acts to fuse the bones of the spine together, the condition is called ankylosing spondylitis or Marie Strumpell disease. The spine typically bows out in the thoracic or chest region, but is flattened in the lumbar region or middle back. This condition causes stiffness and limits the patient's mobility.

Patients with this disease should do therapeutic exercise before the spine becomes completely fused. Therapeutic exercise can help keep the unaffected joints mobile. As long as the condition has not advanced to the point of non-reversibility, exercise may be able to help the patient regain some mobility in the affected areas. However, if the spine has already completely fused, therapeutic exercise can't help.

The exercises should focus on training the muscles of the abdomen, shoulders and hips. Improving these muscles can partially compensate for the inadequate function of the spine.

If you have this condition, you should not

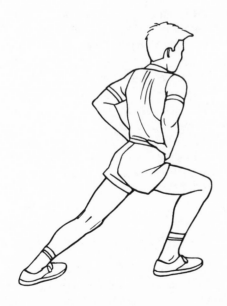

Figure 112. *For hip and knee flexibility*

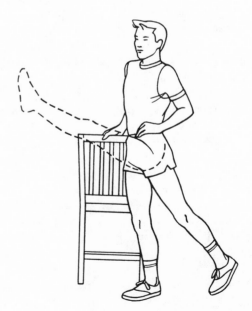

Figure 113. *Leg swinging*

do exercises that will force your spine to bend, extend or twist. You should only do relaxing exercises that are not pain-inducing.

Since this disease limits chest movement, patients are likely to have weak breathing. Therefore, exercises that encourage abdominal breathing and expand the chest region are particularly useful.

If you suffer from ankylosing spondylitis or if you simply want to help strengthen your spine, you should start with some lying-on-your-back abdominal breathing. (Complete instructions are on page 46.) Then do these exercises:

1. As you lie on your back with your hands behind your head, bend your legs at the knees and draw them toward your abdomen. Then raise your feet up with some force. Relax and lower them.

2. Stretch out on your bed with your arms over your head. Then use the momentum of bringing your arms forward to help you raise yourself to a sitting position.

3. As you lie face down, extend your arms to the sides and then lift them up over your back as if you were flying.

4. Standing with your hands on your hips, bend your head forward and backward, then turn it from side to side.

5. Standing with your hands on your hips lean your body gently right, then left.

Each of these exercises may be repeated 10 times or more, as often as twice a day.

Healing Arthritis of the Shoulder

Many people over 40 years old, particularly those with chronic diseases, are bothered by painful and stiff shoulder joints. Inadequate metabolism and generally weakened condition may be partly to blame, according to Chinese medical thought.

The shoulder joints often feel as if they were glued together. While being examined, they may reveal some tenderness. X-rays may also show that both the tendons and bursae (the pads that are supposed to prevent friction) are undergoing calcification. This condition is called bursitis or tendonitis, and it causes inflammation in the tissues around joints.

Physical exercise can frequently help relieve arthritic shoulders. And it can also help prevent the type of bursitis caused by metabolic problems and general physical weakness from ever occurring.

The exercises used to prevent bursitis are relatively simple, but they must be peformed at least once every day and preferably twice. One popular exercise to prevent this unpleasant condition is shoulder rotation. With your arms hanging loosely, you simply make circles beside your body with your shoulders. Do one shoulder at a time—forward 20 circles and then backward 20.

Then put the back of your hand against the front of that hand's shoulder. Push your hand out as if you were pushing something away from you. Do this with each arm 10 to 20 times.

Next, lace your fingers together and stretch your hands high over your head. Lower them behind your head. Do this 10 to 20 times.

To finish up, swing your arms, one forward and one back, like pendulums. Swing vigorously and rhythmically 10 to 20 times.

Freeing Frozen Shoulders

Advanced bursitis of the shoulder can cause so much stiffness and so limit mobility that the patient may feel as if the joint has been frozen. In fact, the condition is sometimes called frozen shoulder. Depending on how severe the disease is, healing exercises can sometimes help defrost those joints.

If the bursitis is caused by an external injury, physical therapy should be used with relaxation exercises. If the condition is due to chronic strain—inflammation of a muscle due to overuse of the upper arm—massage, physical therapy and the appropriate healing exercises are suitable. But if the condition has been brought on by physical weakness, then exercise is the first recourse. Physical therapy and massage should be used, too.

Here is a popular Chinese exercise for pain-

ful shoulder joints. You can select part of it or do the whole set, depending on your strength and flexibility.

1. Stand in a relaxed posture, holding an exercise rod (or wooden stick) in both hands in front of you. Forcefully raise your arms straight out and over your head. (See Fig. 114.) Repeat 10 to 20 times.

2. Holding an exercise rod in both hands straight out in front of your chest, turn from side to side. Let the rod define as large a portion of a circle around your body as possible. Swing particularly hard to the affected side 10 to 20 times. (See Fig. 115.)

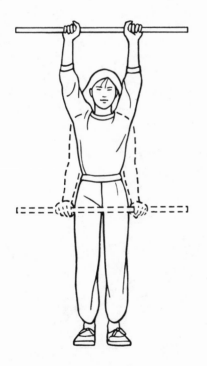

Figure 114. *Using an exercise rod*

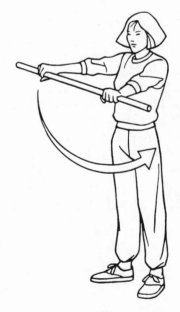

Figure 115. *Twisting with an exercise rod*

3. Stand comfortably with an exercise rod held in both hands behind your body. Raise your arms hard 10 to 20 times. (See Fig. 116.)

4. While standing, raise the elbow of the affected arm as high as you can and touch the back of your neck with your hand without bending your back. (See Fig. 117.) Repeat several times.

5. While standing, reach behind your waist and then raise your hand as far up your spine as possible. (See Fig. 118.) Alternate with your other hand and repeat at least 10 times.

6. While standing, lace your fingers together behind your neck. Turn your elbows as far to the back as possible, as if you were trying to touch them together. Repeat several times.

7. Standing up straight, lace your fingers together and place your hands, palms facing out, against the back of your waist. Now raise your hands as high up your back as possible before returning them to your waist. Repeat this exercise several times without bending your body. (See Fig. 119.)

8. Standing under an exercise pulley, pull on each side, in turn, as shown in Fig. 120.

9. Standing in front of a wall, ladder or tree, place the hand of the affected arm on the object and gradually move it higher. (See Fig. 121.)

10. If you have an exercise wheel available (most Y's have them), turn it with your affected arm.

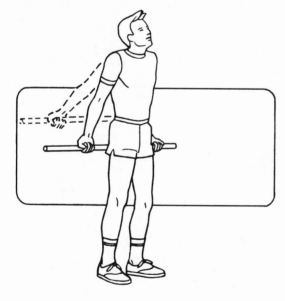

Figure 116. *Lifting with an exercise rod to help heal bursitis*

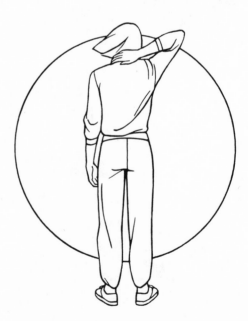

Figure 117. *An exercise to heal shoulder stiffness*

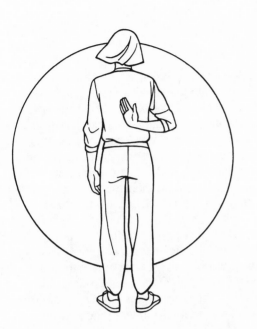

Figure 118. *Reaching high on the back*

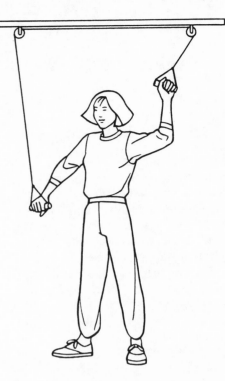

Figure 120. *Using an exercise pulley*

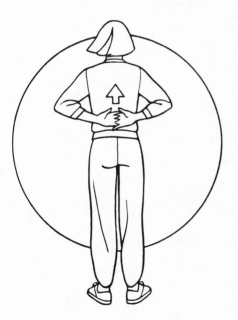

Figure 119. *Raising both arms behind the back*

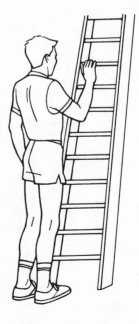

Figure 121. *Touching high on the ladder*

Exercises for Low Back Pain

Lumbago or pain in the lower back is only a symptom, not a disease in itself. The causes of lumbago can be quite varied. One of the most common types—functional lumbago—is mainly a result of incorrect posture or weak muscles of the back and the loin. It's not caused by arthritis, disk problems or sprained muscles.

Functional lumbago can be prevented by engaging in therapeutic exercises. Posture-induced lumbago is brought about by an exaggerated forward curve in the lumbar region of the spine. When a person has this curve, the stress on the vertebrae may cause inflammation and result in pain.

Another type of functional lumbago, found more frequently in the elderly or the physically inactive, is caused by weak muscles of the back and loin. Both abdominal muscles and muscles of the back lack the strength and resiliency to support the lumbar vertebrae in bearing the weight of the body. People with this condition who must sit, stand or walk in the same position for a prolonged period of time often get backaches. Carrying heavy objects or bending their backs is difficult for these people. Their weak muscles force the ligaments and joints of the lumbar vertebrae to carry too great a share of the burden. As a result, painful lumbago develops.

Exercise, if done properly, helps prevent lumbago because it encourages proper posture

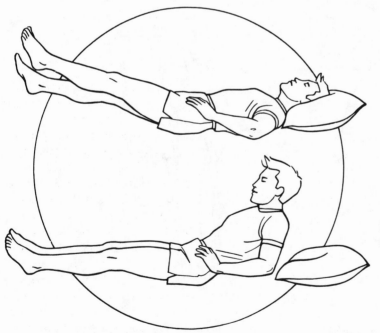

Figure 122. *Partial sit-up for lumbago*

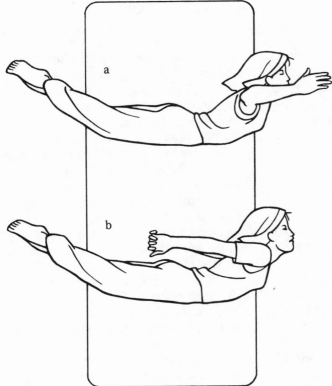

Figure 123. *Building strength in the lower back*

and strengthens the muscles in the abdomen, loin and back. Strong muscles in these areas and correct posture are essential to supporting the spine. Persons who frequently bend their backs in heavy work or strenuous exercise should do preventive exercises even if their back muscles are well developed.

These exercises have proved their value in preventing lumbago. If they cause pain, stop immediately.

1. While lying on your back, lift your legs to an angle of about 90 degrees. Move your legs slightly to your left side and lower them slowly. Raise them again, but this time move them slightly to the right and lower them. Repeat several times.

2. While lying on your back, lift your legs approximately 45 degrees and do a scissors kick in the air until your muscles tire. Rest a minute and repeat this sequence 3 or 4 times.

3. Lie on your back with your hands on your hips. Do a partial sit-up, raising your head and shoulders off the bed. (See Fig. 122.)

4. Lie face down with your elbows bent, your upper arms parallel to your shoulders, and your hands above your head. Raise both upper body and your arms and legs off the bed and hold this posture. Repeat several times. (See Fig. 123a.)

5. As you lie face down, clasp your hands and place them in the small of your back. Draw your body into the shape of a bow by lifting both your upper body and your legs. (See Fig. 123b.)

6. While lying face down, alternately lift one leg at a time.

EDITOR'S NOTE: Since some of these exercises require breath holding and muscle tensing, they may not be suitable for elderly people who have hardening of the arteries or high blood pressure.

Healing Loin Strains with Exercise

When the loin muscles are sprained, the sacro-spinalis muscle, which extends the vertebral column, is usually involved, too.

Muscle injury may result from a sprain or a pull. If untreated, the bleeding and leaking of other fluids can make fibrous tissue form. The fibrous tissue can trigger pain during muscle contractions. The bleeding and excessive fluid secreted after a muscle strain can itself put pressure on nerve endings and cause pain.

Strained muscles can be greatly helped by massage. Applied soon after the injury, massage can lessen swelling and relieve bruising by improving blood circulation. Later, massage can still help even if hard fiber has formed in the muscle. The mechanical action of massage can not only ease the tightness of the scar tissue but also can facilitate its breakdown by bringing more blood to the area.

A medical professional can be called on or the patient can perform self-massage. Described here are three common techniques:

1. While sitting down, rub the scar or the painful spot with the joint of your index finger. Then press, tap and knead the same spot with the thumb. Massage each painful spot 5 to 10 minutes.

2. Sit down and rub your palms together to create some warmth. Then press the affected spot very hard with your palms. Rub the area up and down briskly for 3 to 5 minutes.

3. While sitting, tap and strike your back up and down, either with your palms or with loose fists for 3 to 5 minutes.

The strain of either one of the psoas muscles —loin muscles—can restrict the movement of the spine. Pain, tightness and spasm keep you from using your back.

Exercises designed for treating this condition focus primarily on relaxing the muscles of the loin and the lower back and increasing mobility in the spine. Exercises that involve tensing the muscles of the loin should be avoided.

The following introduces a group of exercises used successfully for treating strained loin muscles. You may select part of the group or perform the whole set. Each exercise should be repeated 10 times.

1. Lying on your back, bend your knees and draw your legs to your abdomen. Hold your knees with both hands to press your back firmly against the bed. Keep the muscles of the loin and the muscles of the lower back relaxed. (See Fig. 124.)

2. While lying on your back with your arms at your sides, lift one leg at a time. (See Fig. 125.)

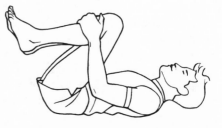

Figure 124. *Pulling knees toward chest*

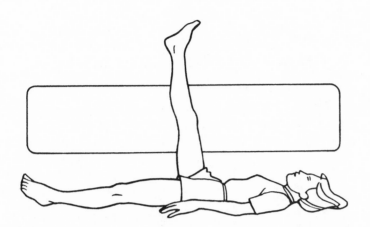

Figure 125. *Leg lift*

Figure 126. *Strengthening the abdomen*

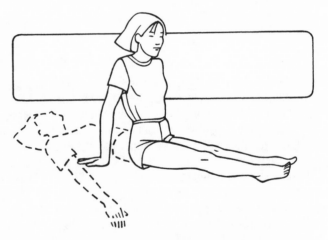

Your movements should be quick but unstressed, and they should not cause pain.

3. From a lying-on-your-back position, sit up straight. You can lean on your arms for support if necessary. Do not bend your body past a 90-degree angle with your legs. (See Fig. 126.)

4. Standing with your hands on your hips, turn your body quickly to the left, then to the right. As you turn, fling your arm out and up in the direction you're turning and let your eyes follow your outstretched palm. (See Fig. 127.) Let your hand circle around and return to your hip as you turn in the other direction and stretch out the other arm.

5. Perform a slow, lunging step with your foreleg bent and your back leg straight. Hold. Switch legs.

6. Standing with your feet apart, clasp your

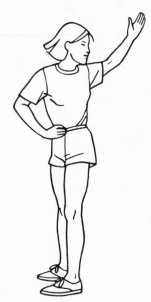

Figure 127. *Turning body and flinging hands*

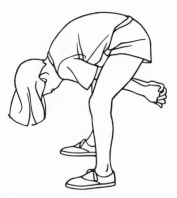

Figure 128. *Splitting wood*

hands and lean forward as though you were splitting wood and following all the way through your legs. (See Fig. 128.) Your motion should be easy and loose, and it should not cause pain.

7. Standing with your feet apart, place your hands in the small of your back. Feel the motion in that area as you twist first to the left and then to the right.

8. The last step is to massage your back and your waist area using the techniques described on page 167.

If you faithfully perform this set of exercises 10 times each, at least 4 times a day, you should note marked relief in no more than a month.

Preventing Knee Strain

Knee strain is a common problem. In its early stages you may feel a weakness and fragility in the knee joint even though you can still engage in physical activity. But whenever you extend your leg, relax it and then push the kneecap downward, you feel pain.

If you treat the problem at this stage, it can be improved relatively easily. Unfortunately, most people do not seek treatment until the condition has worsened and the joint has become swollen. As this deterioration occurs, the patient usually feels a painful soreness below the kneecap. But the symptoms may fluctuate from mild to extremely painful, depending on activity, temperature and other factors. At this stage, if you press your hand against the kneecap and move it around, the friction will be audible and the sensation painful. Pain may also be triggered merely by contracting the quadriceps muscle of the thigh, the muscle most important in straightening the leg. If the condition is serious and of long duration the quadriceps muscle may even have atrophied through disuse.

One expert reported that forming a 150-degree angle with the knee would cause the most friction and pain when the quadriceps contracted. But in China, it has been determined that the most painful angle for those with patella problems is between 110 and 135 degrees. The importance of this fact will be seen in the exercises designed to help heal this problem.

Many people have tried exercise, but obtained no relief. They were left with the impression that there was very little they could do toward alleviating their problem. This view is incorrect. As a matter of fact, there are new techniques, and now much can be done toward improving this condition.

Patients who have shied away from exercise or other physical activities because they feared that exercise might aggravate the pain or worsen their condition have actually slowed down their healing. Lack of physical activity inevitably leads to shrinkage of the leg muscles. That affects joint stability and tissue metabolism. The patient simply becomes more prone to further injury and confounds the existing problems.

Knee strain is usually caused by accidental excessive pressure on the knee. It happens most often when sufficient care is not taken. It is certainly better to avoid this injury altogether if possible than to try to repair it once it occurs. One of the most important preventative measures is proper training methods for athletes, who are frequent victims of knee strain. A good warmup before strenuous exercise, particularly of the quadriceps muscle, is essential. Failure to adhere to a recommended orderly training program can invite this problem. Too much running up and down hills or abrupt stopping after fast running may also cause it.

Exercise, if done properly, can improve the blood supply to the muscles and to the regenerative and connective tissues surrounding the kneecap. An improvement in the metabolic processes in the cartilage, bone and muscle results.

Some people have tried exercise therapy for a period of time for this problem and have experienced lessened pain. But if you find pain and swelling make exercise uncomfortable, external medicine may be used to soothe the pain and reduce the swelling. You may then proceed with exercise.

Healing Exercises for Knee Strain

What types of exercise should be used to treat knee strain? First of all, avoid any movement that causes painful friction between the kneecap and the thigh bone. That is, do not bend your knee at an angle between 105 and 150 degrees.

Another thing that can help is gentle exercise of the quadriceps muscle, the major extensor muscle in the front of the thigh and the muscle most closely connected to the kneecap. This assists in stabilizing the condition. The combination of exercise and deep breathing also can help lessen pain and prolong exercise time. Massage can improve muscle elasticity and expandability and help prevent shrinkage. And massage can be performed anytime—before, during or after exercise. But if you use the forceful knocking technique (described later in this chapter) it is better to do it during or toward the end of the exercise.

The following are several exercises that may be selected based on your condition. As long as you avoid friction between the kneecap and the femur, any exercises designed to strengthen the muscles and ligaments in the knee joint are beneficial. Exercise 2, page 167, is the easiest to do if you want to start simply.

Knocking at the Gate of Life

1. Stand with your feet a shoulder width apart and approximately 1½ feet in front of a wall. Lean your back against the wall and squat down until your shins and thighs form a 90-degree angle. Let your shoulders relax and hang naturally. Try to maintain this position until your muscles tingle.

When your strength has grown, you can move your feet in a bit so that the angle at your knees is approximately 80 degrees. In this position, raise your buttocks slightly without lifting your heels off the ground. (See Fig. 129.) After 1 to 4 minutes in this position, you should feel warmth in your quadriceps muscle. The time to stop this exercise is when your muscle becomes tremulous and it hurts too much to continue.

Walk around for a little while and then repeat this squat 2 or 3 times.

2. This exercise is called the horse-step posture. Stand up with your feet parallel to each other—the distance between them is about 3 times the length of your foot. Grasp the ground firmly with your toes. Squat down halfway so that your thighs and shins form a right angle. Make your hands into tight fists and hold them, fingers up, in front of your waist. Standing up straight, breathe in and out deeply and slowly. (See Fig. 130.) Do this exercise for a few minutes when you're beginning, but extend the time gradually as your condition permits.

When you have gained sufficient physical strength, you can also do the following upper

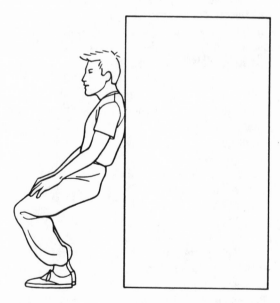

Figure 129. *A good exercise for knees*

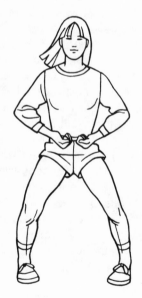

Figure 130. *The horse-step posture*

arm exercises in the same stance:

1. Raise your left fist in a semicircle to the left side up to a position straight over your head while breathing in deeply. Lower your hand through the same half circle to your left thigh while breathing out fully. Breathe in and out several times.

Return your left fist to the original position in front of your waist and lift and lower your right fist in the same manner. Then perform the same exercise with both arms simultaneously.

2. In the same horse-step posture, interlace your fingers, turn your palms away from you and push both your hands out to the front while breathing in and out deeply. Then turn your palms toward you and draw them back near to your chin as you bend forward from the

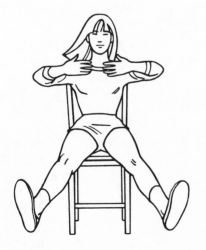

Figure 131. *Building the quadriceps*

waist in a slight bow, breathing out deeply. Hold this position as you breathe in and out fully several times.

3. While sitting on a sturdy stool or chair, lift your legs and hold them off the floor slightly farther apart than your shoulders. Your toes should point up and your feet be at right angles with your legs. Your knees are straight. Hold your arms in front of your chest as if they were wrapped around a large tree. (See Fig. 131.) If you lack the strength for this exercise, you can leave your heels on the ground and use your quadriceps muscle to draw your kneecaps upward. Alternately tense and relax your quadriceps.

4. The kidney and waist strengthening posture starts with you standing with your feet parallel to each other slightly more than a shoulder width apart. It is basically a self-massage. Keeping your legs straight, reach around and rub and press with a downward motion in the small-of-the-back area all the way to the end of your spine. (See Fig. 132a.) Rub the sides of your hips and bend forward as you massage down the outer side of your legs and feet. (See Fig. 132b.) Circle your rubbing along the outer edges of your feet and toes, and then massage the inner edges of your feet. Then massage upward along the side of your legs until your hands reach your knees. Then carefully but repeatedly strike, knock and knead around your knees and the quadriceps muscle on the front of your thigh. As you straighten up, finish massaging your legs. Work up to your abdomen. (See Fig. 132c.) When your hands have reached the navel area, continue the massage around your sides until they return to the starting place in the area of the lower back. Repeat this sequence several times. Do not bend your knees nor tense your quadriceps muscle. Relax as much as possible.

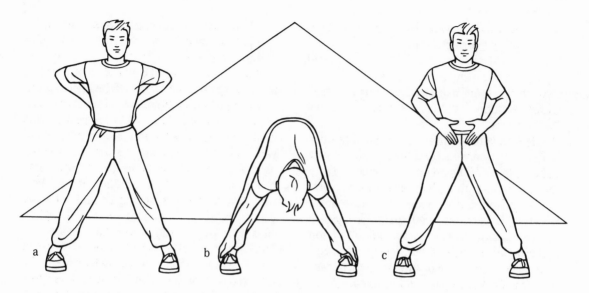

Figure 132. *Waist- and kidney-strengthening massage*

More on Knee Strain

It is important to prevent knee strain. Because of failure to take preventive measures, many fine athletes have hurt their knees and impaired their performance. To stop this happening, teachers or coaches should keep their training plan reasonable and base it on the athletes' sex, age, skill and strength. The exercises for young or female athletes, for instance, need not be as demanding as those for adult men. When an athlete's training is disrupted due to injury to one leg, care should be taken that overcompensation by the healthy leg doesn't result in an injury to the good knee. Before starting the actual exercise, you should warm up. Try to avoid running on a too-hard field that can put excessive pressure on the knee joints. Athletes should wear shoes with adequate bottom cushioning to reduce impact.

The use of spongy material in shoes to absorb shock has significantly reduced the incidence of knee strain in athletic competitions. But attention to strengthening those muscles around the knee as part of the training program is still important in helping prevent strain.

Knee protection devices minimize the impact of sudden shocks on the knees. But prolonged use of these devices may hinder blood circulation. Better protection can be achieved by strenghening the muscles and ligaments in the knee joint area.

Keep the knees warm and protected from wind and moisture. Clean your shoes and socks frequently. Attention to these little things can sharply reduce the possibility of developing knee problems.

Healing Shoulder and Neck Pain

Cervical disk syndrome frequently affects the elderly. Its symptoms include pain and stiffness in the regions of the head, neck, shoulders and back. These symptoms may be aggravated by bending or rotating the head. At times, the pain seems to radiate from the neck to the shoulder and arm, restricting the movement of the cervical vertebrae. Some people's neck movements may have become so restricted their neck muscles have shrunk. These symptoms occur because of arthritis and the protrusion of cervical intervertebral disks creating pressure on the spinal nerve roots and triggering the symptoms of pain and stiffness.

Cervical disk syndrome is treated by pressure release techniques such as traction, neck pulling and massage, by removing aggravating factors such as inflammation and swelling with medicine and physical therapy, by suppressing pain with the same methods and by restoring movement of the head and neck with therapeutic exercise.

Healing exercise not only helps increase the range of motion of the head, neck and back but also strengthens the muscles in these areas. It improves blood circulation and lessens inflammation. Combined with physical therapy, massage and extension it can provide great help.

In the early stage of the disease, therapeutic exercise should be used primarily as a supplement to other forms of therapy. Once recovery has begun, it should become the primary therapy.

Healing exercise for cervical disk syndrome consists mainly of head-turning exercises, which include bending the head forward and backward, turning the head to the left and right, bending the head to the side and rotating the head. The most emphasis should be placed on the first two exercises. Perform these 10 to 15 minutes at a time, 3 or 4 times a day. Your movements should be slow and even, and they should not cause pain. Do not make hard abrupt moves. When you have reached the maximum stretch, hold this position for 1 minute. This will build up muscular strength as well as help lengthen shrunken muscles and ligaments.

One more thing needs attention. If cervical spondylosis—collapse of the vertebrae—is the cause of cervical disk syndrome, it is quite probable that the spine that supports the chest and lower back—the thoracic and lumbar vertebrae—may also be affected. In this case, exercises should be directed at strengthening the entire spine. If the disease results from arthritis of the back of the cervical vertebrae, exercises designed to correct the abnormal curvature of the thoracic spine should also be performed, such as those starting on page 172.

Here is a suggested progression of exercises for the head and neck. Remember to do them slowly and easily. Start with just 1 to 4 repetitions. Work up to more, but stop whenever you are tired.

1. While sitting, slowly turn your head from the right to the left and back again.

2. While sitting, bend your head forward, your chin pointing to your chest. Then bend your head backward and look up.

3. As you sit, tilt your head to the right and raise your face toward the ceiling. Feel the stretch from your jaw to your neck. Then tilt your head to the left and do the same thing.

4. Let your head roll slowly in a complete circle, then reverse directions.

Sometimes the muscles in your neck and shoulders may be so tense that they affect the movement of the head. If so, add this exercise to your routine. First hunch one shoulder toward your ear, and then the other. After you have alternated shoulders for a while, raise both shoulders simultaneously until the tension has eased.

Correcting Rounded Shoulders

Physically inactive individuals who read, write or sew in sitting positions for long periods of time are more inclined than average to develop rounded shoulders. The nature of their work requires that their arms be continuously in front of their bodies. As time passes, the major muscle of the chest, the pectoral, shrinks while the major shoulder muscle of the back, the trapezius, becomes slack and weak. As a result, the shoulders turn inward and slant down. To prevent this, people who do this kind of work should make a point of doing exercises designed to expand the chest muscles.

To help correct rounded shoulders that have already developed, perform the following exercises:

1. While standing, touch your fingertips to the rear of your neck and draw your elbows as far to the rear as possible. Keep your head high. Hold this position for several minutes before relaxing.

2. Touch your hands together in front of your shoulders, then swing your elbows to the rear to expand your chest. Repeat several times.

Some people have protruding shoulder

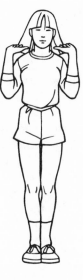

Figure 133. *Thrusting the chest forward*

blades that resemble chickens' and birds' wings. These people are said to have winglike scapulae. Their problem is caused by weakening of the anterior serratus muscle which fails to hold the scapulae in proper position.

The following exercises can be used to correct this condition. First let your arms just hang down naturally as you stand in a comfortable position. Then lift your hands, palms up and fingers back, to a position just above your shoulders. Now thrust your chest forward and try to make your shoulder blades touch. (See Fig. 133.) Hold as long as you can.

Exercises for Flatfeet

Flatfeet is a condition in which the entire sole comes into contact with the ground when the person stands. (See Fig. 134.) People with flatfeet have very low or flattened arches.

Not all flat-footed people need to do corrective exercises. Some flatfeet may produce no unpleasant symptoms. According to a survey conducted in China, about 25 to 49 percent of students and 12 to 40 percent of the athletes were flat-footed. But flatfeet did not affect the athletes' ability to jump or any other aspect of their athletic performance. Flatfeet with no accompanying symptoms may simply be an anatomical characteristic and not a disorder. Since it does not bring about other problems, there's no need to correct it.

The typical case of flatfeet does have symptoms, though.

The condition may hinder blood circulation in the lower legs, bring pain to the sole of the foot and induce fatigue during walking. A flat-footed person often has muscles and ligaments in the feet that are weak and loose. In severe cases, bones may protrude, Chinese doctors say. This type of flatfeet may be caused by muscle weakness resulting from physical inactivity in childhood and adolescence.

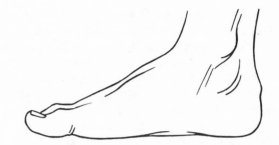

Figure 134. *Flatfoot*

The cause may also be the abnormal development of bones, ligaments and muscles, or an incorrect walking posture in which the big toes turn outward excessively and the person tends to walk on the inner edges of the feet. Or an infectious disease may have weakened the arches and foot muscles.

Therapeutic gymnastics are effective in correcting flatfeet if they are used in childhood or adolescence. Adults unfortunately will get less pronounced results.

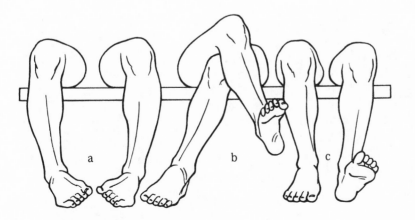

Figure 135. *Exercises to build arches*

The exercises should focus on training certain muscle groups in the lower leg—including the flexor digitorum longus, the anterior tibial muscle and the posterior tibial muscle—as well as the muscles of the foot. The following exercises have been chosen for correcting flatfeet. Do them as many times as feels good.

1. While sitting in a chair, turn your big toes in and roll your feet onto their outer edges. (See Fig. 135a.)

2. While sitting with your legs crossed, bend your top foot up while you alternately curl and raise your toes. (See Fig. 135b.)

3. While sitting down, keep one heel on the ground and flex your foot back. (See Fig. 135c.) In this position, curl and then extend your toes.

4. While sitting, spread your toes and then bring them together. Repeat this many times.

5. While sitting, use your toes to grasp a small object such as a pencil, marble, or piece of cloth, or use your toes to put dried peas or marbles in a bowl as in Fig. 136a.

6. While sitting, manipulate and roll a ping pong ball, a small rubber ball or a tennis ball between the soles of your feet as in Fig. 136b.

7. Walk on a specially designed, sturdy board shaped like an inverted V, one foot on each side.

8. Walk on your tiptoes.

9. Walk on the outer edges of your feet.

10. Walk on the outer edges of your feet with your toes curled.

11. Walk on a gravel path, beach or uneven road.

Anyone whose flatfeet are spasmodic should not do these exercises. If they cause you pain, you should stop doing them, too. But flat-footed people usually need more exercise, not less. If you have flatfeet you may have weak hip, thigh, abdomen and lower leg muscles, and you should do exercises that will strengthen not only those areas, but your whole body.

Exercise and Spinal Curvature

At the turn of this century, a scientist observed that though the lizard slithered as it crawled, its spine always grew very straight. The scientist

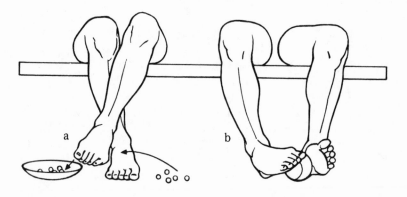

Figure 136. *Grasping objects to build arches*

attributed the absence of spinal curvature in lizards to the twisting of their spines as they crawled. Inspired by this discovery, a set of crawling exercises for children was developed to help correct spines that had unnatural bends to the side. One of these exercises is shown in Fig. 137.

This crawling exercise is, however, no longer widely practiced. It has been largely replaced by newer and superior corrective exercises.

These exercises have definite value in correcting curvature of the spine to one side. Before discussing these exercises, let's talk about the causes of scoliosis—the name given to spinal curvature to either side.

A normal spine is straight up and down and doesn't curve to either side. When scoliosis occurs, it may be one of two types: either sickle-shaped (or C-shaped) curvature—the spine curves only to one side—or snake-shaped (or S-shaped) curvature—the upper and lower sections of the spine curve to opposite sides.

Scoliosis can also be classified by causes. The type that doctors call rachitic scoliosis results from the disease of malnutrition called rickets, caused by a deficiency of vitamin D in the diet. Underdeveloped bones and muscles compounded by poor posture and prolonged sitting are responsible for the damage in this type of scoliosis. Another type results from tilting the pelvis for a long period of time. The most common causes of this pelvic misplacement are a misdistribution of body weight to one side while sitting, an inequality in the length of the legs or one leg being weaker than the other— usually because of polio or other serious illness. In these circumstances, the pelvis is forced into an unnaturally crooked position. Ultimately, the patient develops scoliosis.

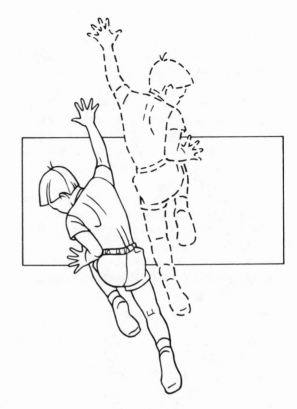

Figure 137. *A lizard exercise for bent spines*

The last type is habitual scoliosis. Some children develop lateral curvature of their spines as a result of incorrect reading and writing postures in which they slant their heads and upper bodies to one side.

These three types of lateral curvature occur most frequently during childhood and adolescence. Therefore, prevention should begin in the early years. It's important first to eliminate contributing factors—to help the child develop a proper standing and sitting posture. Children should also be encouraged to be physically active so that they will increase muscle strength and develop fitness. Strong muscles and ligaments help hold the spine in its proper position.

Once it's noticed, scoliosis should be treated as early as possible. Corrective exercises are more effective for children and adolescents than for adults. The extent to which they'll help will depend on the degree of curvature.

First-degree lateral curvature is the least serious. It is seen only after the child has been sitting or standing for a long time. The curvature disappears when the patient hangs in space from an overhead horizontal bar. This kind of curvature is caused by muscle weakness, and it can be easily corrected. The patient should engage in

healing exercise to strengthen the back muscles and prevent the condition from getting worse.

Second-degree lateral curvature is more serious. The bend has become more permanent. The patient can no longer make it disappear when hanging from a bar. But this condition can still be helped by therapeutic exercise.

Because of its effects on muscles, ligaments, bones and cartilage, third-degree lateral curvature is quite serious. In addition to the sideways curve of their spines, some patients may suffer from hunchback and a twisted thorax, which may impede the functioning of their hearts. At this stage, therapeutic exercises cannot be of much help.

In exercises for correcting scoliosis, stretch-

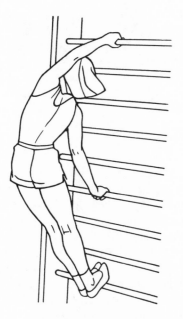

Figure 138. *Bending on portable gym*

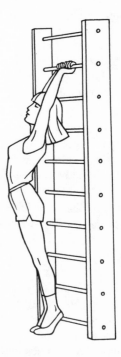

Figure 139. *Stretching on portable gym*

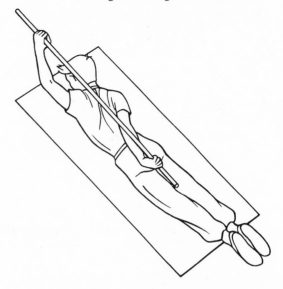

ing the spine and toning up the back muscles are the primary focus. It is also the purpose of the exercises to strengthen overstrained and weakened muscles caused by a convex curvature and to stretch shrunken muscles caused by a concave curvature.

Here's an exercise sequence commonly used to help correct S-shaped curvature. Do each only until you feel slightly tired.

1. Facing a portable gym, reach over your head and grasp a high crossbar with your left hand and a lower one with your right hand. Hang for 3 to 5 minutes. You may take 1 or more breaks as needed during this exercise.

2. With your right hand on your hip, raise your left arm over your head by swinging it up sideways with force.

3. Standing with your arms on your hips, take a long step forward with your left leg. Bend the left leg but leave the right one straight. In this

Figure 141. *Correcting a bent spine with an exercise rod*

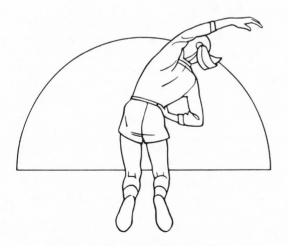

Figure 140. *Bending exercise to heal the spine*

position, stretch your left arm above your head while you reach down forcefully with your right.

4. Stand with your right side near a portable gym. You may stand on a low bar or the floor. Grasp a high bar with your left hand and a bar near your hip with your right. Bend your upper body as shown in Fig. 138.

5. Stand with your back facing the portable gym. Lift your heels from the floor and stretch your body as high as it can go. Get your arms as high up as possible. (See Fig. 139.)

6. Kneel with your hands on your hips. Raise your left arm and bend your upper body to the right. (See Fig. 140.)

7. While lying on your stomach, hold a long exercise bar (or any wooden bar) with your left hand stretched out in front and your right hand stretched down. Raise your head and upper body. (See Fig. 141.)

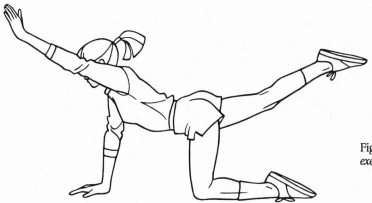

Figure 142. *A graceful exercise for the back*

8. Lie on the right side of your body with a solid type of pillow (or sandbag) under the most protruding part of the curvature.

9. Get down on all fours. With your right palm and left knee on the ground for support, lift your left arm and right leg and extend them. (See Fig. 142.)

10. Lie on your back with your arms at your sides. Inch your way forward, one shoulder at a time, using only your back muscles and shoulder blades.

Exercises for Saddle Back

Lordosis—the medical name for hollow back or saddle back—refers to the condition in which the spine has an excessive curve toward the front. (See Fig.143.)

Lordosis can result from habitual bad posture, from uncorrected post-pregnancy temporary lumbar displacement or simply from weak back muscles.

In children, the condition is frequently caused by a combination of malnutrition and weak muscles, the result of stomach or intestinal disease. These children must be given adequate nutrition as well as corrective exercises.

Except for its unusual appearance, hollow back may not cause other symptoms. However, in the female sex, lordosis frequently causes lumbago, or low back pain. To treat the lumbago, you should attempt to correct the lordosis through exercises. Exercises designed for correcting saddle back focus on stretching muscles in the lower back and strengthening the abdominal muscles. The following four exercises have been selected for saddle back sufferers. Do each as many times as feels good.

1. Sit astraddle a stool with your back against the wall. Pull in your abdomen until your lower back touches the wall.

2. As you sit on the floor or bed with your legs straight out in front of you, pull in your stomach as you did in exercise 1. This is an excellent posture for straightening your hollow back.

3. While lying on your back with your knees bent, raise your feet back and over your head. In this position, bring your legs together and make wheel shapes with your feet by stretching and retracting your legs. The larger the wheels, the better.

4. As you lie on your back with your arms behind your head, raise your legs so that your hip joints are bent at a 90-degree angle. In this position, bend and stretch your legs one after the other as if you were riding on a bicycle.

Exercises 3 and 4 are physically demanding. If you find them too difficult to complete, you may perform other simpler exercises designed to strengthen the abdominal muscles, such as those on page 115.

Exercises for Round Back

Round back refers to the condition in which there is a semicircular protrusion of the upper back. Viewed from the side, a person with round back may be seen to have a protrusive upper spine and forward leaning head and shoulders.

When the condition is mild, it does not appear to affect any physiological processes. When it is serious, it can interfere with breathing and cause upper back pain. (See Fig. 144.)

There are believed to be three types of round back. The adolescent type frequently seen in children and youth may be caused by underdeveloped back muscles, using a desk that is too low, inadequate room illumination and nearsightedness—conditions that force the child to bend forward. It may also be hereditary.

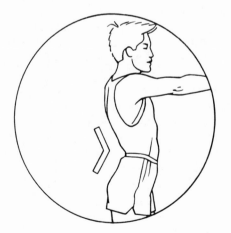

Figure 143. *Saddle back*

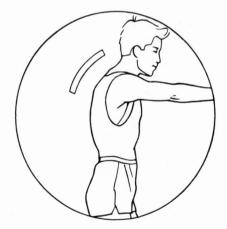

Figure 144. *Round back*

Occupationally induced round back occurs when a person's job demands too much forward bending. In the elderly, round back may result from an alteration in the tissues of the spinal disks, which in turn weaken back muscles. The spinal column no longer receives proper support and the thoracic vertebrae curve toward the back.

It's important to prevent the adolescent type by using tables and desks of the right height, providing adequate light in classrooms and reading rooms and encouraging children to participate in physical exercise.

But when round back does occur, it can be corrected through healing exercise. These strengthen the back muscles, stretch the trunk and expand the thorax. Gymnastics, swimming and certain hanging exercises are also helpful.

The following describes a frequently used series of corrective exercises. You may repeat the entire sequence as many times as you like.

1. Stand with your legs together and extend both arms out in front of you. Then swing them to the rear as forcefully as you can. Take a nice stretch and then do it again.

2. While standing with your legs together, lace your fingers behind your back. Then stand on tiptoes and raise your arms as you arch your back and thrust your chest forward.

3. While standing with your legs together and an exercise bar (or any wooden bar) in your hands in front of you, lift your arms with sufficient force to stretch your trunk.

4. Stand up with your legs together and an exercise bar held in both hands behind your back at the shoulder blade level as shown in Fig. 145a. Turn your body left and right as you stretch your trunk.

5. Standing with your feet apart, hold an exercise bar behind your shoulder blades as you

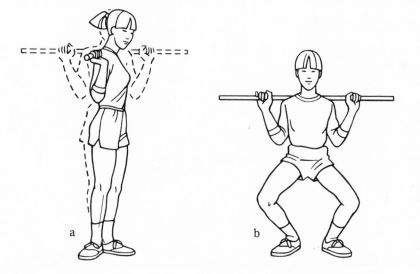

Figure 145. *Healing round back*

a   b

did before. Squat halfway down while keeping your back straight. (See Fig. 145b.)

6. Stand facing a portable gym with your legs together. Raise your arms to grasp a high crossbar. Lean forward, arching your back and thrusting your chest forward.

Pigeon Breast and Exercise

If you look carefully at the breast of a chicken, you will see that its breastbone or sternum juts sharply forward like the spine of a wooden boat. Some people have chests that resemble those of pigeons or chickens. Their breastbones stick out and the sides of their chests are slightly sunken. This condition is frequently referred to as pigeon or chicken breast.

Pigeon breast is formed in early childhood. Because of chronic tonsillitis or other obstructions to the airways some children develop respiratory problems. They cannot breathe in enough air, nor does their thorax expand as it does in normal children. Their ribs fail to form a natural bend. As time goes by, these children become pigeon-breasted. Young children who suffer from rickets, a disease of malnutrition, are also prone to developing pigeon breast due to underdeveloped bones.

If the deformity is slight, pigeon breast may return to normal by itself as the child gets older. If it's serious, the abnormality may become permanent.

Children who have pigeon breast are susceptible to bronchitis and pneumonia because of their weak lungs and inefficient breathing.

Work should be done to correct their problem as early as possible.

Children with pigeon breast should be examined by a physician. If their problem is related to chronic tonsillitis, therapy should involve clearing the respiratory tract of infection. These children should also be taught to practice deep breathing with emphasis on training in proper inhaling. They should practice breathing in through the nose and out through the mouth.

If their condition is caused by rickets, they should be given plenty of vitamin D in nutritional supplements and should be encouraged to exercise where they can get plenty of sunlight and clean air.

Corrective gymnastics and exercises can definitely benefit children with pigeon breast. Here are some exercises that can expand the chest, strengthen respiration, and thus, normalize the chest.

Use dumbbells to strengthen your chest muscles by raising small weights from your sides to shoulder level. You can also swing your arms forward and backward either with or without a dumbbell in your hand—or make circles beside your body, again with or without dumbbells. Running, jumping, swimming or playing basketball are also recommended.

By the time of late adolescence and adulthood, pigeon breast has become permanent. It can no longer be corrected. But individuals with this problem can still strengthen their chest muscles and improve their breathing with the preceding exercises.

CHAPTER EIGHT

Healing the Genito-Urinary System

康

Healthier babies, a fast delivery and a speedy recovery from childbirth are just a few of the benefits of Chinese exercises for the genito-urinary system.

And when problems do develop in these important areas of the body, the Chinese have exercises to help put things right. By increasing and regulating energy flow, stimulating circulation, building flexibility, strength and resiliency, these exercises can make getting better easier and faster.

And all of these techniques can be used to help protect and care for ourselves and to avoid costly and painful health problems before they start.

Exercise for an Easier Pregnancy and Birth

Thanks to the evolutionary process, human beings have acquired the ability to walk on two limbs instead of all four. This ability has not been gained without a price, however. Part of that price is that the soft tissues that make up the pelvic floor must now absorb pressure exerted by the weight of the entire upper body. Upright walking also makes it more difficult for venous blood to return to the heart. To add to these problems, there is a tendency to overlook exercise for this part of the body. This is especially true for sedentary types whose jobs require them to remain stationary for long periods of time. The result for women is that pregnancy and labor may overstrain and weaken the muscles of the pelvic floor and the abdominal wall. The uterus and vagina may prolapse and other internal organs may be displaced downward.

But therapeutic exercise can strengthen the muscles that support internal organs. In addition, it improves circulation in the pelvic cavity, helps keep the heart healthy and reduces chronic inflammation.

Exercises for pregnant women and exercises that will aid women when they go into labor have been widely hailed in recent years. Done correctly and regularly they offer many benefits.

During pregnancy, the body undergoes many changes. For one thing, the presence of the developing fetus limits the movement of the diaphragm, interfering with respiration. Moreover, there is an increasing demand on the circulatory system. Disturbances in metabolism may also occur.

Therapeutic exercise can help improve respiratory and circulatory functions and speed up the metabolic process. In addition, regular exercise can strengthen the diaphragm and abdominal muscles, making for an easier labor and a smoother delivery.

And exercise begun 12 to 16 hours following the birth can help restore physical strength and speed up the tightening of overstretched muscles in the new mother's abdominal cavity and pelvic floor.

Clinical studies have shown that women who engaged regularly in exercise after giving birth were less likely to develop prolapses. It also took less time for their uteruses to contract back to their normal shape and for their urinary and bowel functions to return to normal. And, as is discussed in more detail in this chapter's section on prolapse, healing exercise can speed up recovery from that condition, especially if it is performed shortly after the birth.

Pregnant women should also exercise to benefit their unborn child. Studies have shown that expectant mothers who are physically inactive —who don't even walk very much, sometimes out of fear—are more likely to give birth to children who are less healthy than babies of active mothers. Babies of inactive mothers also have been shown to be more likely to develop heart diseases.

Therapeutic exercise can help women with many problems related to their sex organs. It can heal or help heal prolapse of the uterus, prolapse of the vagina, chronic pelvic inflammatory disease, bladder incontinence, tilting of the uterus, painful menstruation, symptoms associated with menopause or abnormal menstruation due to organic factors. Exercise should not be performed, however, by anyone with acute inflammation of the reproductive organs, a high fever, pelvic abscess, malignant tumor, excessive bleeding or an extrauterine (ectopic) pregnancy.

Exercises for Pregnancy

Pregnant women should learn the technique of deep breathing to ease their pregnancy and the process of labor. Deep breathing, if done correctly, will not only help improve overall body tone, but also will speed up delivery. It can also improve the elasticity of the abdominal and pelvic muscles and the flexibility of the hip joints. All of these can contribute to an easier and safer delivery.

The first trimester of pregnancy is the riskiest for miscarriage because the fertilized egg has not yet firmly implanted into the uterine wall. Women who have histories of miscarriage should not excercise during this period. Most pregnant women, however, will have no problem with occasional short-distance walking or performing deep breathing. Relaxation breathing exercises also may help lessen any problem with nausea, vomiting or loss of appetite.

The following set of exercises is recommended for women between the fourth and sixth months of pregnancy. You can do all the exercises in one session or only a few at a time. Remember that your movements should be slow and soft, and they should not cause fatigue.

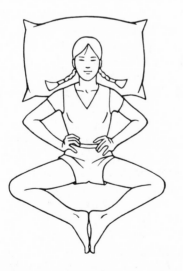

Figure 146. *Exercising for an easier pregnancy*

1. Do this exercise right after waking in the morning. Lie on your back with your legs stretched out, your arms at your sides. Perform grasping and scratching motions with your hands and feet 50 to 100 times.

2. While lying on your back with your legs naturally extended and your arms comfortably alongside your body, first roll your arms inward and outward 50 times. Then do the same with your legs 50 to 100 times.

3. Lie on your back with your legs straight out and together. Bend your knees and draw your feet up to your buttocks. Lift your pelvis while constricting your anus. Then lower your pelvis slowly and relax your anus. When your hips are on the bed, face the soles of your feet toward each other and slowly relax your thigh muscles so that your knees spread as wide as possible. (See Fig. 146.) Breathe in and out deeply 3 times. Then extend your legs to their full length. Repeat this exercise 10 to 20 times.

4. Lie on your back in the shape of a cross, your arms straight out to the sides. Trying to keep your hips still, reach across your body with your right hand to touch the left, which shouldn't move. Turn to the other side in the same manner. Touch each hand 10 or more times.

5. While lying on your back with your legs naturally extended, tense and relax your anal and vulval muscles 30 to 50 times. Try to coordinate this exercise with your breathing rhythm — inhale while tensing and exhale while relaxing.

6. Standing with your arms on your hips, take a long step forward to form an arch. Your front leg should be bent and your back leg straight. Repeat 4 to 8 times with each leg.

7. Stand with your hands on your hips. Without bending your knee, lift your left heel off the ground. Alternate with the other heel. Do this 4 to 8 times for each foot.

8. Stand with your hands on your hips and lift each knee as high as you can, one after the other. Do this 4 to 8 times per knee.

9. While standing on one leg, turn the other foot around in circles, fully stretching the ankle. Do the same with the other foot. Repeat this sequence 4 to 8 times.

If it's difficult to keep your balance, you may hold onto an object for support while doing the last three exercises.

From the seventh month of pregnancy to the time of delivery, the body weight of the expectant mother increases so much that the center of gravity shifts toward the front. Because it is difficult to maintain balance during this stage, the pregnant mother should concentrate on exercises that are performed on her back. To avoid fatigue, the amount of exercise may be reduced, particularly during the last month of pregnancy.

Healing Exercises for After the Baby

The process of childbirth takes a toll on the mother's resources. After the birth, the new mother may feel tired and weak for some time. Her stomach and intestines aren't functioning as well as they should, and the muscles of her pelvic floor and abdominal region are slack.

Therapeutic exercises after childbirth can shorten the time required for recuperation. They strengthen both abdominal and pelvic floor muscles. In addition, they speed up the return of the uterus to it's pre-pregnancy state. And they help restore the normal workings of the stomach and intestines. Only in the case of certain diseases should new mothers avoid exercise. When there is fever, bleeding, kidney disease, liver disease,

active tuberculosis, cardiovascular system disease, abnormal metabolism or there has been a Caesarian section exercise should not be undertaken. But generally if the delivery is smooth, the new mother can begin exercise within 12 to 16 hours after childbirth.

Two sets of exercises follow. You can select whichever you like for practice. Increase or decrease the number of repetitions, depending on your strength and recovery. How often you practice may also be determined on an individual basis. After the first month, you can add additional exercises from the group for treating prolapse of the uterus.

1. While lying on your back with your arms at your sides, slowly lift your arms straight up in the air as you inhale. Lower your arms as you exhale.

2. While lying on your back, raise one leg with the knee bent, then lower it. Alternate with the other leg.

3. Lie on your back with your legs bent and knees raised. Lift your hips from the bed, then lower them.

4. While lying on the left side of your body, bend and lift your right leg, then lower it. Turn over and repeat with the other leg.

5. While lying on your stomach, bend your knees and bring your heels as close as possible to your buttocks. Lower them.

6. Lie on your back with your knees bent and do sit-ups. If it's difficult at first, you can use your arms for support. Later do it without holding onto anything.

7. Lie on your back and pretend to ride a bicycle.

Exercises 1, 2 and 3 can be performed the day after delivery. Exercises 1, 2, 3 and 4 can be done on the third day, and 1, 2, 3, 4, 5 and 6 on the fourth day. From the fifth to seventh day, the entire set may be performed. In the beginning, repeat each exercise 4 to 6 times. Later on, increase to 8 to 12 repetitions.

More Post-Delivery Exercises

1. Lie on your back with your legs naturally stretched out and your arms at your sides. Slowly perform grasping and scratching motions with your hands and feet 50 to 100 times.

2. Lie on your back with your legs naturally extended and your arms at your sides. Constrict your anus as you breathe in, and relax it while breathing out. Repeat 5 to 7 times.

3. While lying on your back with your legs stretched out and your arms at the sides, bend your knees and draw your heels toward your buttocks as you breathe in deeply. Then let your feet slide back down until your legs are fully extended as you breathe out deeply. Repeat 3 to 7 times.

4. Lying on your back with your knees drawn up and bent, your heels touching your buttocks and your hands under your head, lift your hips off the bed as you breathe in deeply. Your weight should be on your shoulders and the soles of your feet.

Breathe out deeply as you lower your hips. Then constrict your anus while breathing in and relax it while breathing out. Repeat this 3 to 7 times.

5. Lie on your back with your arms at your sides. Draw your hands up along your sides, bending your elbows. Continue raising your hands across your shoulders and up behind your head as you inhale. Exhale as you draw your arms back down. Repeat 3 to 7 times.

6. While lying on your stomach, inhale and draw your legs up to the sides, knees bent. Exhale and slowly stretch your legs back out. This exercise can usually be performed 4 to 5 days after delivery. It's good for helping to prevent backward tilting on the uterus—which may be aggravated by prolonged lying on your back.

How Healing Exercise Can Help Painful Periods

Dysmenorrhea refers to pain that occurs just before or at the onset of menstruation. The pain, which may be cramplike, is centered in the lower abdomen.

There are two types of dysmenorrhea. Primary dysmenorrhea affects young women who are having their first periods. Psychological factors, weak abdominal muscles, an underdeveloped or misplaced uterus may all have a role in causing this problem. Secondary dysmenorrhea is usually caused by gynecological disorders such as an inflammation of the reproductive organs.

Therapeutic exercise works better for primary dysmenorrhea. It can improve blood circulation in the pelvic cavity, strengthen abdominal muscles and contribute to an improved mental state.

According to scientific studies, healing exercise has relieved or cured painful periods of between 25 and 85 percent of the female students who tried it.

The healing exercises used in treating dysmenorrhea are designed to increase movement in the abdomen and to improve blood circulation in the pelvic cavity. The following exercises are easy to do and have proven therapeutic value. The exercises can be performed 2 or 3 times a day before or at the onset of menstruation.

1. Lie face up with your legs bent and knees raised. Perform abdominal breathing about 10 times, feeling your abdomen slowly inflate like a balloon and then slowly fall.

2. Stand up with your hands holding the back of a chair. Without bending your legs, lift and lower first one heel and then the other. Do this about 20 times.

3. Holding onto the back of a chair as before, do 5 deep knee bends.

4. While lying on your back, lift and bring your knees up to touch your chin. Do this about 10 times.

The Muscles of the Pelvic Floor

The muscles of the pelvic floor, also known as the pelvic diaphragm, collectively comprise the levator ani muscle. The levator ani muscle includes the pubococcygeus, iliococcygeus and sacrococcygeal muscles, of which the pubococcygeus muscle is the largest and the strongest. The pubococcygeus muscle interlaces with the sphincter muscle of the urethra, the outlet of the tube leading from the bladder, and inserts into the vaginal sphincter, a circle-shaped contracting muscle.

The levator ani muscle serves two important functions. It supports the organs inside the pelvic cavity and constricts the lower end of the rectum and the vagina. It is also closely related to the sphincter muscle of the urinary bladder and the sphincter muscle of the urethra.

The muscles of the pelvic floor are frequently blamed when prolapse of the anus, the rectum or the uterus occurs, and for incontinence of urine. To treat these diseases, it is necessary to strengthen the weak and malfunctioning muscles.

This can be accomplished by training the muscles in the regions of the anus, abdomen and hip.

The following exercises will prove especially helpful. Do them each several times, until you feel mildly fatigued.

1. While lying on your back and breathing in, lift your hips slightly and constrict the muscles of the pelvic floor—it should feel like trying to hold back a bowel movement. Breathe out as you relax the muscle.

2. As you lie on your back with your legs bent, breathe in and lift the sacral region—your lower back—constricting your buttocks, hip and pelvic floor muscles as in exercise 1. Let go slowly and relax back onto the bed. Relax your entire body.

3. Lie on your back with your legs full length but crossed at the ankles. Place your feet against a wall. While breathing in, tighten the muscles of the pelvic floor and lift just your lower back—the sacral region—from the bed. Next, lift both your head and your hips slightly as you breathe in. Relax your entire body as you breathe out.

4. Lie on your back with your legs drawn up and bent. Press your knees against each other as hard as possible while raising your pelvis. Relax your thighs and lower your pelvis.

5. Sit on a low stool with your legs stretched out but crossed at the ankles. Press your knees together as hard as possible while tightening the muscles of the pelvic floor.

6. Kneel on your hands and knees. Arch your lumbar vertebrae—the midback—in a raised curve and constrict the muscles of the pelvic floor as you breathe in. Relax your back while breathing out.

7. Squat with your buttocks resting on your heels. As you inhale, tighten both your hip,

buttock and pelvic floor muscles, then lean forward and put your hands on the floor, assuming a kneeling position. Return to the squat while breathing out.

8. Sit on a high stool and constrict the muscles in your pelvic floor, lifting your feet from the floor and breathing in. Relax and lower your feet as you breathe out.

Of the preceding eight exercises, the first is the most important. In fact, you can do this exercise alone and still expect good results. Practice it 2 or 3 times a day for 15-minute or 20-minute sessions, or do it 200 times in a row.

Healing a Prolapsed Uterus

Prolapse of the uterus is caused when pelvic ligaments become so slack that the womb displaces downward into the vagina.

This condition can be treated with healing exercise. To be effective, however, the patient must have a positive attitude and believe that the disease can be cured and that therapeutic exercise can make a difference. Clinical studies have shown that systematic training of the levator ani muscle has enabled many patients with slack abdominal walls or muscle tears that occurred during labor not only to strengthen the muscles and ligaments that support the pelvis but to partially or completely cure their prolapse. Moreover, symptoms associated with prolapse of the uterus—backaches, soreness near the waist, heavy sensations in the pelvic cavity, difficulty urinating, abnormal menstruation and protrusion outside the vagina have often disappeared before the complete retraction of the uterus was achieved.

If the prolapse is serious, treatment should begin with lessening the inflammation and swelling. After these conditions have been corrected, the uterus should be lifted manually and held in place with a pessary—a device used to support the uterus. To consolidate this temporary effect, the patient should begin participating in therapeutic exercise on a regular basis. Experience shows that therapeutic exercise can effectively treat first-degree and second-degree prolapse, and it is also satisfactory for third-degree prolapse. (In first-degree prolapse, the cervix has descended into the lower vagina. When it's a second-degree prolapse, the cervix protrudes outside the vagina. In the third-degree, the uterus itself protrudes.) Here are several good exercises. Select a few that you like for practice.

1. This is a postural exercise. Lying either face up or face down, raise and support your hips with a cushion. This position will speed up the process of retracting the uterus. After the uterus has retracted, tense the muscles of the pelvic floor as if you were trying to keep yourself from urinating or moving your bowels. Tense and relax these muscles 100 to 300 times each practice session and do 2 to 6 sessions a day. This technique is easy to carry out and is especially appropriate for patients who are at the early stage of third-degree prolapse. After recovery or toward the end of recovery, you no longer need to support the buttocks with a cushion each time. You can do the exercise in any comfortable position, including sitting and standing.

2. Lie flat on your back. Relax each and every part of your body completely. With your hands beside your body, bend your knees and draw your heels close to your buttocks. Supporting yourself with your feet and shoulders, lift your hips off the bed while breathing in. Lower your hips as you breathe out. Constrict your anus while breathing in. Relax your anus and your entire body while breathing out. Do this 10 to 30 times.

3. After your uterus has returned to its proper position, you can do this exercise. It can be performed standing or lying down on your stomach, back or side. With your legs fully extended and crossed, constrict both your anus and vulva as hard as possible. Then relax the muscles of your legs and pelvic area completely. Repeat 100 to 300 times. After you've become used to this tensing-relaxing cycle, you can practice constricting your lower pelvic muscles as you breathe in and relaxing them while breathing out.

4. Lie on your back with your hands on your thighs. Without using your elbows, raise the upper portion of your body into a sitting position as you simultaneously constrict both your anus and vulva. Then lie back down slowly and relax your entire body. Repeat 10 to 30 times.

5. Lie on your back in the shape of a cross with your arms out to the sides and your palms up. Then without moving your left hand, roll your upper body and slap your left palm with your right hand. Try not to move your hips. Slap your right palm with your left palm in the same manner. Do this 10 to 30 times.

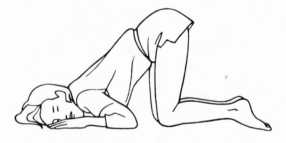

Figure 147. *An exercise to heal a fallen uterus*

6. Kneel on a bed. Lower your shoulders and head to rest on the bed while leaving your hips in the air. Your thighs should be perpendicular to the surface of the bed. (See Fig. 147.) In the beginning, maintain this position for 5 minutes, once in the morning and once in the afternoon. Gradually increase each session to 20 minutes. This exercise is very helpful to patients with a backward tilting uterus, a common problem in patients suffering from prolapse of the uterus or vagina. After recovery from a prolapse, this exercise will keep the uterus in good condition.

Pelvic Inflammatory Disease and Therapeutic Exercise

Among the symptoms of chronic pelvic disease are backache, lower abdominal pain, pain near the base of the spine, a thick, white vaginal discharge and abnormal menstruation. A pelvic examination may reveal abnormal thickenings, tenderness and lumps. Women with evidence of acute inflammation or pelvic abscess should not exercise. But in its chronic state, the disease can be helped by healing exercise.

The purposes of therapeutic exercise are to improve blood circulation and reduce chronic inflammation. Several useful exercises are described here.

1. As you lie on your back, relax, concentrate and press gently with your thumb against *Kuan Yuan*, the acupuncture point located 3 inches below your navel. (See Fig. 148.) Rub and knead lightly around this spot first clockwise then counterclockwise, 300 or more times in each direction. After practicing this exercise for an extended period of time, you may experience a sensation of warmth and a feeling that your

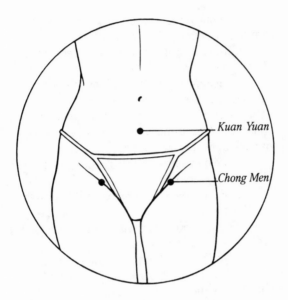

Figure 148. *The* Kuan Yuan *and* Chong Men *points*

internal organs are moving in the same direction as your thumb. Do this exercise in the morning and afternoon.

2. Lying on your back with your legs stretched out naturally, press hard, with your thumbs or middle fingers, around *Chong Men*, the acupuncture points located between your thighs and groin and just over the femoral artery. (See Fig. 148.) Silently take your pulse to the count of 30 or 40, then release the press. After resting for 1 minute or so, resume pressing and counting on the other side. Do this sequence 3 times. If you have varicose veins, you should not perform this exercise.

3. Now do an exercise and breathing technique. Sit quietly on the very edge of a chair. With your palms resting on your lower abdomen

and your legs apart, breathe in and out deeply one time. While breathing out, bend your upper body forward until your head is lower than your knees. At the same time, press hard against your lower abdomen with both hands. This will cause the abdominal pressure to increase and your diaphragm to ascend. Allow as much residual air as possible to escape. Then release your abdomen, stretch your neck forward and raise your head slowly as you breathe in deeply and peacefully, sitting gradually back up to your original position. Repeat this process 7 to 14 times. Then stand up and march in place for a few steps. To finish up, do 6 or 7 deep knee bends.

4. The last exercise is walking around a circle taking large steps. Start with a circle as large as 6 feet in diameter. Later you may grad-

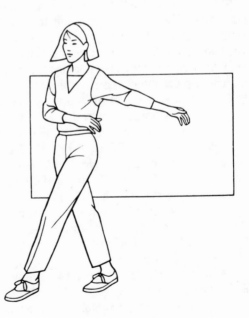

Figure 149. *Walking with swaying arms*

ually reduce it to about 3 feet. Your arms may hang naturally or you can swing them from side to side. As your left foot steps forward, sway your arms to the left. (See Fig. 149.) As your right foot steps forward, sway your arms to the right. If you feel dizzy, circle in the opposite direction. Walk 10 to 20 minutes a day. If you feel dizzy or uncomfortable and changing directions doesn't help, you may walk in a straight line instead.

Healing Cystitis

Cystitis is the most common bladder disorder. Its symptoms include frequent and painful urination and passage of pus or blood with the urine. Sometimes chronic cystitis symptoms are mild and may even be overlooked.

In chronic cystitis, the inflammation may affect part or all of the mucous membrane. The areas most frequently affected are the lower triangular portion and the outlet of the bladder, the trigon and the neck. Chronic cystitis is a stubborn disease that resists treatment.

But regular showering or bathing in a mineral spring bath can have some healing effects. Regular exercise over an extended period can also be of therapeutic value. In China, some patients who practiced *Pa Kua Ch'ang* (The Palm of the Eight Diagrams) and *Hsing I Chuan* (The Fist of Form and Will) for 1 year cured diseases of nearly 20 years duration.

However, people who have acute cystitis—the severe, active form of the disease—should not exercise. They should take plenty of rest, and of course, have medical care.

Chronic cystitis may respond favorably to the following healing exercises. You may do each as many times as feels comfortable unless directed otherwise.

1. While lying on your back with your legs naturally extended and about 2 feet apart, turn your feet out and in to cause your legs to roll slightly from side to side.

2. Lie on your back with your legs drawn up and your feet close to your buttocks. Raise your hips as high into the air as possible as you breathe in deeply. Lower your hips as you breathe out.

3. Lie on your back and ride an imaginary bicycle.

4. Lie on your back with your legs straight up. Cross your legs back and forth over each other. (See Fig. 150.) Then with your legs crossed, draw small circles in the air.

5. While standing in a natural posture, rub and push on the region around your tailbone with both hands for a few minutes. Knock this area hard 30 or more times with one fist. Then standing with your legs together, breathe in

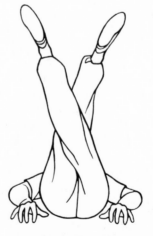

Figure 150. *Leg crossing and circling*

deeply and squat down as low as you can. Wrap your arms around your knees and squeeze as you breathe out fully. Repeat 6 or 7 times. If you want more of a workout, the exercises for silicosis patients starting on page 102 are appropriate.

Exercises for Prostatitis and Vesiculitis

Patients with chronic prostatitis, an inflammation of the prostate gland, tend also to suffer from chronic vesiculitis, inflammation of the seminal vesicles.

Some men don't even notice the symptoms of these diseases, but others are more sensitive to them. Some men experience pain, usually in their lower backs, buttocks, pelvic floors, groins or sex organs. They may also feel it in their lower abdomens and legs. If the inflammation is long-standing, the patient may also suffer headaches and dizziness. If the condition gets worse, the patient may not be able to sit long because of the pain in the lower back and pelvic areas.

Prostatitis may also cause frequent and painful urination and a feeling that the bladder is not empty. The urethra may sting and burn. Sometimes the patient may notice white secretions coming from the urethra. These are signs of an inflamed prostate and typically appear when the patient gets out of bed or after he has a bowel movement. Premature ejaculation, impotence, a loss of sexual desire and nocturnal emissions may also occur.

No totally satisfactory treatment of chronic prostatitis and vesiculitis has yet been found. In recent years, the use of a comprehensive approach, combining traditional Chinese medicine with Western medicine, therapeutic exercises and warm water baths of 10 to 20 minutes each

night has proved helpful in alleviating the symptoms. Both *Tai Chi*, the Supreme Ultimate Exercise, and *Nei Yang Kung*, the internally nourishing *Ch'i Kung* breathing technique (see page 49), have proved effective. The following exercises are also helpful:

1. In China, this is called a buttock-vibrating exercise. Lie on your back with your legs naturally extended. Alternately tighten and relax your buttocks as fast as you can so that your hips jiggle up and down. Repeat this until your muscles are tired. The aim of this exercise is to loosen your pelvis and get the energy moving there.

2. Lie on your back with your legs drawn up and your feet near your buttocks. Using your shoulders and feet for support, lift your hips high off the bed, constrict your anus and breathe in deeply. Then let go suddenly and allow your hips to drop to the bed to further vibrate your pelvic area. As your hips fall, relax your entire

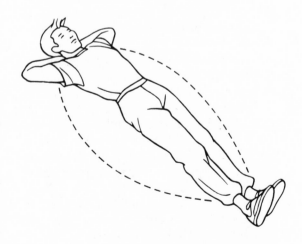

Figure 151. *The goldfish exercise*

body and breathe out deeply. Repeat this sequence 10 to 20 times.

3. The goldfish exercise calls for you to lie on your back with your legs naturally extended and to sway your waist from side to side like a fish swimming in the water. (See Fig. 151.) Repeat 100 to 200 times. You may also do the same exercise on your stomach. This is especially effective for treating constipation and abdominal bloating.

4. To do the fanning exercise, lie on your back, lift your legs 40 to 45 degrees off the bed and fan and cross your legs 50 to 100 times.

5. The bicycling exercise—lying on your back and pedaling—should be done at least 50 to 100 times.

6. The kidney- and waist-strengthening exercise is a self-massage combined with a stretch. Stand with your feet slightly more than a shoulder width apart. Rub around your navel with both hands. Continue rubbing around the sides of your waist to the small of your back and your tailbone. Bend forward and massage down the outer sides of your legs, around your feet and up the insides of your legs until your hands are back at the starting point near your navel. Repeat this process 20 or 30 times.

7. Stand naturally with your feet a shoulder width apart and make loose fists with your hands. Turn your body from side to side using the lumbar vertebrae in the small of your back as the axis. As you turn to the left, knock your lower abdomen with your right fist, and your tailbone with your left. (An illustration showing a man doing this exercise is on page 54.) Repeat as many times as you wish.

8. To perform the can-lifting exercise you will need to prepare a relatively simple piece of equipment. Find a wooden rod that is 1½ to 2 inches thick and as wide as your shoulders. Drill a hole in the middle of the rod. Tie one end of a string firmly to the rod through the hole and tie the other end to a can or a brick weighing no more than 5 pounds. To begin the exercise, stand as if you were riding a horse, legs widely set, knees bent and toes firmly clutching the ground. Hold the rod straight in front of you, one hand on each end, and your "tigers' mouths"—the space between your thumbs and forefingers—facing each other. Now use your hands to roll the string up until the can or brick is at chest level. Release the string and lower the object slowly. Repeat this exercise several times. The weight of the can and the number of times you perform the exercise may be increased gradually as your condition improves. After doing this exercise, knock or strike your arms, chest and abdomen with loose fists or your palm to give yourself a massage and stimulate your circulation.

Exercises for Varicocele

Varicocele—a varicosity of the network of veins that lies along the spermatic cord—occurs most often on the left side of the bodies of 20-year-old to 30-year-old males. In most cases, the condition is not even noticed until discovered during a medical examination.

Varicocele rarely needs special medical treatment unless it impairs sperm production or causes swelling, pain or a feeling of downward displacement. The condition may improve on its own in some young patients after they marry. But swellings or lumps in the genital area should be evaluated by a doctor.

In cases of varicocele, it's generally recommended that patients move their bowels regularly and avoid chronic constipation. This practice will minimize the possibility that waste matter will increase pressure on the left spermatic veins, hindering the return of blood to the heart.

Also useful is washing the area with cold water. This will cause the spermatic veins to constrict and reduce blood congestion in the veins.

If varicocele symptoms are troublesome, you can also relieve them by wearing a supporter or a tight brief.

These suggestions may also help: take a cold water bath or, as previously suggested, wash the scrotum with cold water daily. The best healing exercises are those designed to strengthen the muscles in your abdominal walls and to facilitate blood circulation in the pelvic cavity.

These exercises are usually performed on your back, and not only facilitate intestinal movement, but also reduce blood congestion in the veins in the pelvic cavity. For these reasons, they prevent constipation and alleviate varicocele symptoms. The exercises described in the section dealing with habitual constipation (see page 111) as well as exercises that are used to strengthen the muscles of the pelvic floor (page 186) are appropriate for treating varicocele.

Varicocele patients should not do strenuous exercises. Long-distance running, weight lifting, soccer, basketball and similar sports may cause dilation in the veins and aggravate the symptoms.

Index

Page numbers in *italic* indicate illustrations.
Page numbers with a *t* indicate tables.